MY MOST INTIMATE
SECRETS

MY MOST INTIMATE
SECRETS

The path to eternal youth

Mark Mounier's

Library of Congress Control Number: 2014915965
ISBN: Hardcover   978-1-4633-9186-7
                        Softcover   978-1-4633-9185-0
                        eBook   978-1-4633-9184-3

Print information available on the last page.

Rev. date: 19/02/2015

To order additional copies of this book, please contact:
Palibrio
1663 Liberty Drive
Suite 200
Bloomington, IN 47403
Toll Free from the U.S.A 877.407.5847
Toll Free from Mexico 01.800.288.2243
Toll Free from Spain 900.866.949
From other International locations +1.812.671.9757
Fax: 01.812.355.1576
orders@palibrio.com
521784

CONTENTS

CREDITS...7

SPECIAL COLLABORATORS..9

INTRODUCTION...11

SPECIAL THANKS 13

DEDICATION 15

PREFACE..17

PART 1
A YOUNG AND BEAUTIFUL APPEARANCE

CHAPTER 1. Nutrition 21

CHAPTER 2. Hair Care..27

CHAPTER 3. Skin Care 35

CHAPTER 4. The Importance of Eyebrow and Eyelash Care 41

CHAPTER 5. The Magic of Having and Maintaining Enviable Lips 45

CHAPTER 6. Dental Care 47

CHAPTER 7. The Secrets to Makeup................................49

CHPATER 8. Bust Care...57

CHAPTER 9. Feet and Hand Care....................................61

CHAPTER 10. Care of Elbows and Knees.........................67

CHAPTER 11. Prevention and Treatment of Stretch Marks 69

CHAPTER 12. Tips and Tricks for Cellulite 71

CHAPTER 13. My Ten Most Intimate Secrets....................73

PART II
MY MOST INTIMATE SECRETS

CHAPTER 14. Life Plan 87
CHAPTER 15. Attitude/Aptitude..91
CHAPTER 16. Love...95
CHAPTER 17. Love and parents...101
CHAPTER 18. Love towards our Mother 103
CHAPTER 19. Love towards our Father 109
CHAPTER 20. Love towards our children 113
CHAPTER 21. Love towards Siblings..117
CHAPTER 22. Love towards our grandparents..123
CHAPTER 23. Love towards Friends..129
CHAPTER 24. Love towards our Partner 133
CHAPTER 25. Forgiveness...139
CHAPTER 26. Love and the Universe..141
CHAPTER 27. Quotes, Thoughts and Phrases
    That Have Impacted My Life 147

Farewell...151
Dear Brother Mark..153
MY GREATEST GIFTS..155

CREDITS

DRAFTING & CONSULTING:
César Cedillo

**COVER PHOTOGRAPHY
DESIGN:**
Hugo Salgado & Fernando Rocha
Jonathon Franco & Roy Vega

HAIR & MAKE-UP:
Fernando Hernández

GRAPHIC DESIGN & EDITORIAL:
José Carlo Velázquez Almada

SPECIAL COLLABORATORS

Gustavo B. Moreno de Dios
(Dental surgeon and orthodontist)

Martha Rosa Moreno de Dios
(Attorney at law)

Melissa Almada Moreno
(Psychologist-Specialist on Psychoanalysis)

Wynidy Almada Moreno
(Physical therapy and rehabilitation)

Rossy Diaz
(Fashion design and producer)

Sandra Diaz lazo
(Liberal arts)

Antonio Parra Sepulveda
(International business)

Brandon Robinson
(Aeronautical engineer)

Marco Colom
(Book coordinator)

Martin Ortiz
(TV producer and public relation)

INTRODUCTION

Hi! It's your friend Mark Mounier's. I'm very excited to reach you through this medium, making you my accomplice and partner in this wonderful dream becoming reality. This book was in the making for many years through professional studies, and through daily personal practices and experiences. My commitment to this project is the result of years of a compilation of beauty issues, resolved on a basis of elementary and practical procedures with immediate results, substantiated on the true problems that involve all human beings that desire a beautiful and youthful appearance.

In this book you will be able to find recipes that are not only practical and economical, but also easy to prepare with ingredients found in your own kitchen. You will also learn the beneficial properties of all these ingredients, obtaining better results when mixing them together.

With all this, you will be lead to the right path for obtaining a spectacular head of hair and skin as smooth as a peach.

We will talk about dieting and its correct definition, how to guide yourself while following a diet and the steps you should take to begin an accurate diet.

You will learn about the importance of caring for hands and feet, which are the very important parts of our body.

I will give you the hottest tips on applying makeup, so you may obtain the same results as a model featured on the cover of a magazine.

In the exercise chapter, I will guide you towards fun and easy ways to execute routines that bring surprising results (if you follow the steps exactly as instructed).

These are a few things that you will find beneficial along with other beneficial topics that you will discover as you take this tour. With this said, I would love to wish you all the benefits in the world: success in everything you do and that you accomplish becoming the person you have dreamed of through **My Most Intimate Secrets**.

SPECIAL THANKS

To my clients and friends who have motivated me to realize this dream.

To my co-workers for contributing. I will take this opportunity to thank all these people who have always believed in me on every project that I have realized.

To my celebrity friends for sharing their most intimate secrets on how to look like the hottest stars in Hollywood.

To all those friends who throughout my professional career and personal life have given me their unconditional support, especially my group *Por siempre amigos (Forever Friends)*, who have shared moments of my life since childhood until today.

To my dear friend and coworker, Fernando Hernández, who kept reminding me that I had been working on this book for years, and insisting that I bring it to life.

I am infinitely grateful to a dear friend who has been my collaborator to be able to fulfill this work, Cesar Cedillo.

DEDICATION

I dedicate this book entirely to my family, for all their support, help and unconditional love:

Lorena Moreno, Mark Angelo Moreno and Victoria Cecille Moreno.

To my parents, Mr. Luis and Mrs. María de la Luz Moreno.

Finally, my special dedication and infinite gratefulness to that Universal Being who has always been holding my hand to take me to the path of success and guide me through life up until today.

PREFACE

From a very young age Mark Mounier's showed interest in the world of aesthetics, earning a scholarship in the prestigious beauty academy; Vidal Sassoon, highlighted as one of the best students. This started his pattern to become a specialist in the different areas of cosmetology in the most prestigious beauty schools around the world.

In his list of skills he has demonstrated to be not only an expert but also an authority in the world of beauty, therefore, not only capacitating experts around the world and in countries known to be pioneers in the world of aesthetics, but also has been invited to participate in seminars, radio shows and T.V. shows such as: *El show de Christina*, *Sábado Gigante*, *Los Angeles en Vivo*, *Viva el 22* and *Que no te cuenten*, on Mundo Fox network.

He has had the opportunity to work and coexist with great personalities from the world of entertainment such as Salma Hayek, Jennifer López and the International queen of Salsa, Mrs. Celia Cruz, who found in him not only her stylist and makeup artist, but also an endearing friend for many years.

Mark Mounier's has worked as support for companies like Vidal Sassoon, Paul Mitchell, Coca-Cola and Burger King.

He has participated in television commercials, music videos, movies and radio talk shows.

One of his most recent works has been his collaboration with one of the most important international cosmetics companies, capacitating its team in more than 15 states and 25 cities.

Mark Mounier's is known as the image designer to the rich and famous. He also owns his own line of hair care products "My most intimate secrets" as well as his two exclusive fragrances for man and woman.

Mark Mounier's is a restless and innovative human being, a father, a friend and a great entrepreneur with many dreams, projects and surprises to come.

For all these, Mark Mounier's is known as a fundamental pillar in the world of beauty and cosmetology.

PART 1

A YOUNG AND BEAUTIFUL APPEARANCE

CHAPTER 1

Nutrition

We could not start talking about how we can have an exterior beauty without first recognizing and taking into account that beauty starts from the inside out.

For all we know is that everything we eat is manifested onto our exterior and is fully visible, from the look of your hair, the sparkle in your eyes, to your nails and skin.

I suggest that you start by reviewing your diet and making a visit to your primary care physician to develop a perfect meal plan according to your needs.

. . . .
DIET
. . . .

It is extremely funny how the word diet is interpreted as a way to lose weight, when in fact it is not.

The word diet comes from the Greek word δίαιτα, or diaeta, in Latin, which means diet. A diet is food each person consumes in their own different ways.

Often we confuse diets with a special diet for weight loss or to treat certain diseases. The reality is that good or bad, every human being carries out some kind of special diet.

For sure, we can recognize that it's a lifestyle and is influenced by culture and directly affected by social, economic and above all, personal factors.

It is more convenient to visit your doctor, he will probably recommend some clinical analysis, whose results will have the information necessary to determine the type of diet to lose, gain, or simply keep you at an ideal weight.

And most importantly, a safe and healthy way of life.

The Failure of Diets

Frequently, we hear talk of a new diet to lose weight that is in fashion, or that your aunt took part of and it was fabulous. It is important to understand that as human beings our bodies react individually, therefore not all diets will work for us like it does for others to get the same result.

It is not a question of luck, its simple logic and the fact that we are different from others. In no way do I recommend any type of diet which is not under the supervision of a health care professional because you will most likely fail in the majority of cases and in others you could have fatal results.

The Truth about Fad Diets

It is important to remember that if you're overweight today which may bother you, it was not done overnight, so it is impossible to lose it magically over night. This is where my recommendations come in.

The easy road does not lead you to a successful result. All those so-called easy and magical diets to lose weight fast turn out to be a real failure. First, you will not get the desired result, and second, you'll fall into the famous crash diet, bringing as a result the re-gain of the lost weight and very often gain more.

All you will achieve is feeling disappointed and sad. As the famous scientific quote states: "The shortest distance between two points is a straight line".

It's a character flaw when we decide to do a fad diet to lose weight, when a special event or important date is around the corner and then the anxiety takes hold of us in those thirty days or less, forcing us to commit atrocities in order to achieve the weight of a professional model and go against our own health.

Ideal Weight

Ideal weight is the right proportion of your height and age. It is something that we must acknowledge and accept. Once we have recognized it and with the help of a professional, you can carry a discipline that will be consistent with good nutrition, exercises and the ability to achieve the weight that you always wanted.

Now that you know the perfect weapons to achieve that ideal weight with better results, take into consideration that you will follow my directions to the letter to not make any more mistakes.

Finally, let me remind you: your decision, discipline and perseverance will be your best allies!

Exercise

Add life to your life

How many times have we heard health professionals say that exercising will add life to our life? This phrase can confuse us in some ways. Let's clarify: exercising will add quality to our lives, therefore, we must understand that exercising regularly will bring many benefits and will improve the quality of life.

It is very common in my lectures, speaking about exercising, that when asked about this matter, that most people assure me that they don't perform any type of physical activity, even having knowledge of the importance of exercise. But what's most surprising is the number of excuses to prevent such an activity. Some are: "I don't have enough budget to pay for a gym", "The area where I live does not have safe parks or safe areas", and the most common one is: "I have no one who can accompany me".

The importance of exercise is that it is a very valuable weapon that can help us tone our muscles and lose body fat. Exercise fills us with energy, prevents and helps various kinds of physical and mental diseases, such as osteoporosis and depression, just to name a few.

It is well known that many of us resist exercise for different types of reasons, but everything is due to the lack of knowledge about the importance of doing so, and particularly the reluctance and personal motivation.

So to continue I will tell you a secret to achieve the greatest benefits of your exercises: The music.

Fortunately, since the beginning of mankind, music has been a very important part of our day to day routines. So I want to suggest that you start your day with music to your liking and making body movements to physically enhance your morning activities whatever they may be.

It is important to start with soft music, preferably with slow movements, for about 5 to 10 minutes in the first week and change the music gradually to something more rhythmical.

This will also support you to move a little bit more quickly, adding more minutes to your routine. So practice this between the second and third weeks of the month.

Once you've mastered it, I suggest for the first month, you use music that will allow you to make faster movements when doing your household chores and to complete the desired thirty minutes of physical activity as recommended by health professionals.

After accomplishing this goal, you'll get results and the benefits of this type of exercise. You can infect others with your enthusiasm and you will manage to also motivate and encourage others to see the effects you've achieved.

Your family can also be in good physical condition, they will have leaner muscles and probably a better figure, more positive attitudes and will be full of energy. They, like you, will add quality to their lives.

CHAPTER 2

Hair Care

Let's talk hair care! Considering that it's an extension of our skin and as previously mentioned in the first chapter about Nutrition, this will affect and benefit the appearance of your hair in an amazing way.

Let me give you some tips and recipes that will help anyone obtain healthy and shiny hair no matter what hair type.

It's extremely important to know the type of hair you have, be it normal, dry, thick, mixed hair, damaged or just plain fine or thick hair.

Once you've identified your hair type, you should buy the shampoo and conditioner that best suits your hair. (It's recommended that you purchase these products at a Salon because let's face it, you buy cheap you get cheap results.)

I recommend a good hair washing routine, as follows: Get used to washing your hair every other day, in other words leave a day in between.

The importance of this routine is to give your natural oils an opportunity to renew and to be able to travel from root to tip thus ensuring a brilliant shine.

Next, I will show you some recipes using all natural ingredients that you can prepare in the comfort of your own kitchen.

• •

Normal Hair

• •

To keep hair healthy, shiny and youthful, I've come up with the following recipes that you can switch to as desired or needed. You must apply them once a week as part of your washing routine to maintain the beauty of your hair.

Given that people with normal hair are only a lucky few, which surely has to do with their diet and the right choice of a good shampoo and conditioner. Practice and apply these recipes to help you maintain and highlight the natural beauty of your hair.

Recipe 1

Ingredients: 2 teaspoons of olive oil, 2 teaspoons of sweet almond oil, 2 teaspoons of bear oil and a teaspoon of honey

Preparation: In a glass bowl mix all of your oils except for the honey. Place the bowl in the microwave and heat for 5 seconds, just enough to warm up the oils. Once you've removed the bowl from the microwave, add the honey.

Application: Using your fingertips and with the help of a wide tooth comb, this will distribute the mixture evenly from root to tip. Immediately after applying the entire mixture to your scalp and hair, place a shower cap on your head. The natural heat from your scalp will help absorb and benefit the oils and honey onto your hair.

For this treatment, you'll leave on for a period of 20 to 30 minutes. In the meantime, prepare your shower for your first rinse. In a mixing bowl add warm water and juice from two lemons. This will help you cut off excess oils from your scalp. Then proceed to washing your hair with shampoo followed by conditioner as you would do normally.

If you follow this treatment, I can guarantee you that your hair will maintain that normal balance with a more healthy and enviable shine.

Another alternative would be the following recipe:

Recipe 2

Ingredients: 1 whole banana, 1 teaspoon of margarine and a teaspoon of nuts.

Preparation: Add the ingredients into a blender or food processor and mix until you get a paste consistency.

Application: Using your fingertips and a wide tooth comb, evenly distribute the mixture from root to tips. Afterwards place a shower cap over your entire head and leave on for 20 to 30 minutes. In the meantime, prepare your shower for your first meantime: In a mixing bowl add warm water and juice from two lemons.

Next, proceed to wash your hair with shampoo followed by conditioner as you would do normally.

Keep in mind that these two recipes are highly moisturizing and the benefits increase when mixed properly. With these tips you can create your own recipe according to your needs and preferences. Take advantage of it and enjoy the benefits!

. . . .
Dry and Damaged Hair
. . . .

Dry and Damaged hair I assess in multiple ways. The cause could be the result of chemical processes or poor water quality and the bad choice in shampoo and conditioner, thus causing dry and abused hair.

It shouldn't go without saying that it's very important to choose a good shampoo and conditioner specifically for dry and damaged hair.

To continue, let me give you some tips and recipes that will help you with this problem.

Recipe 1

Ingredients: Some Mayonnaise (amount would depend on the length and volume of hair), a shower cap and a wet warm towel

Application: On dry hair apply mayonnaise leaving two inches away from roots and distribute it evenly with your fingertips. Place the shower cap over your head and then wrap the wet warm towel over your head. This will help your hair to absorb in the nutrients from the mayonnaise.

Another good alternative would be:

Recipe 2

Ingredients: A cup of organic yogurt, 2 teaspoons of honey and 6 strawberries

Preparation: Using a blender or food processor, mix all of your ingredients until you get a creamy consistency.

Application: Evenly distribute the mixture from root to tips and leaving it on for 20 to 30 minutes. Then proceed to washing your hair with shampoo followed by conditioner as you would do normally.

Another great effective idea would be:

Recipe 3

Ingredients: 1 box of Jell-O mix (any flavor), a cup of organic yogurt, 2 teaspoons of brown sugar and a spoonful of castor oil

Preparation: Mix all of your ingredients in a bowl.

Application: Apply the entire mixture from root to tips then place a shower cap on and leave it on for 20 to 30 minutes. Then proceed to washing your hair with shampoo followed by conditioner.

Here's some great tips for you: trim your tips at least once a month. For this type of hair, it's important to refrain from the use of dryers, flat irons and any styling tools as much as possible.

Now the frequent use of this recipe depends on how damaged your hair is and for the first use of this recipe, you would just need to do this once a week. As soon as you start to see any healing results then you'll just need to do it once a month thus ensuring good shiny, silky and healthy hair.

· ·

Oily Hair

· ·

I'm going to let you in on a little important secret about people with oily hair, for years they have fallen into the trap of washing their hair too frequently, some do it every day or even two to three times a day. Not knowing how much to clean your hair to fix the problem, all you've done is revived the sebaceous glands, promoting the segregation of a large amount of oils and aggravating the problem of oily hair.

In this case I recommend you to start using the following recipes along with a daily shampoo for a week without using conditioner. Between the first and second week, after the problem is controlled, wash your hair every other day and of course use the right shampoo. Then you could use a conditioner but only using it for your tips.

An excellent tip is to add a teaspoon of Milk of Magnesia to your shampoo to help make the results and benefits more prominent when treating oily hair.

Recipe 1

Ingredients: 4 cups of water and orange peels from 2 oranges

Preparation: Add your ingredients to a saucepan and boil to create the infusion of both the water and orange peels.

Application: After washing your hair with shampoo, rinse your hair out with the orange infusion twice a week until the greasy hair problem is gone.

Recipe 2

Ingredients: Half a cup of apple cider vinegar and 4 cups of water

Preparation: Mix and stir your ingredients at room temperature.

Application: This recipe should be used after washing your hair with shampoo twice a week to fix the problem and then once a month as maintenance.

Recipe 3

Ingredients: 1 potato, 2 cups of water and juice from half a lemon

Preparation: In a pot, add your water and potato and let it cook for 15 minutes. Remove your pot from the heat and then add your juice from the half lemon.

Application: After washing your hair with shampoo, rinse your hair out with the potato water infusion and leave it in for 5 minutes then rinse your hair out with plenty of water.

. . . .

Fine Hair

. . . .

We must remember for certain that there is still no magic solution to help us grow our hair, much less give us more than what we already have but there are some solutions that you can achieve to make your hair look more abundant and healthy.

Recipe 1

Ingredients: 6 carrots, a couple of lettuce leafs and a small bunch of alfalfa sprouts

Preparation: Place your ingredients into a juicer and extract the juices.

Application: Drink it! Drink this juice once a day, twice a week for a month, and then once a month as maintenance.

Recipe 2

Ingredients: A plastic bottle with an atomizer, three-quarters of water by one-fourth part of a dark beer.

Preparation: Pour the ingredients into the plastic bottle, mix by shaking it and place the bottle into your refrigerator.

Application: Whenever you wash your hair, remove excess water with a towel and immediately pull out the bottle from the refrigerator and spray your hair with this recipe.

Recipe 3

(To get voluminous hair)

Ingredients: Half a cup of water and the necessary amount of watercress to form a paste

Preparation: In a blender place and mix your ingredients to obtain the desired consistency, as mentioned before, to a paste.

Application: Place the mixture on your hair evenly leaving it on for 20 minutes. Then rinse with plenty of water, followed by your regular shampoo.

To make your hair appear more abundant, I recommend using a style in which it stays shoulder length. Avoid conditioners and fixatives to give style.

Thick Hair

Thick hair is usually associated with being rebellious and heavy and I have some great solution recipes for it.

Recipe 1

Ingredients: An avocado pulp, a tablespoon of olive oil and one egg yolk

Preparation: With a fork mix these ingredients into a bowl until you get a paste.

Application: Distribute the paste onto your hair evenly and leave it in to act for forty- five minutes.

This procedure should be repeated two times a week for a month. As soon you get your hair to be easier to handle, repeat this treatment once a month.

Also Recommended

Recipe 2

A conditioner bath

Realistically this is a great solution to thick and rebellious hair.

Procedure: Before washing your hair with shampoo, use enough conditioner in your hair to saturate it. Using your fingertips, give your scalp a massage in a circular motion for five minutes, continuing with using shampoo and end by repeating the same procedure by applying conditioner again.

In addition, visit a good stylist that can recommend an appropriate cut to your hair type and for the shape of your face.

CHAPTER 3

Skin Care

Let's begin by knowing that the skin is the largest organ that the human being possesses. The care and maintenance to our skin is very important. That will determine how we prolong and extend a younger and energetic appearance.

· ·

Secrets to Getting a Peach Perfect Skin

· ·

For a less attractive, withered and dull skin, exfoliation is very important to get rid of the dead cells that accumulate on our skin.

One of my most intimate secrets that will help you solve those problems is the following:

Take a half cup of white sugar to your bathroom, moisten your skin with warm water and with your hands take a lot of sugar and rub your entire body with the sugar starting with your face. Give yourself a vigorous massage in a circular motion until the sugar granules are dissolved.

Again take another portion of sugar and repeat the same process on the remaining parts of your body until you reach the feet.

You'll obtain the benefits of exfoliation resulting in a youthful and beautiful appearance with an even skin tone.

Facial Masks

For Dry Skin

Before the application of any mask I recommend washing your face and neck with plain soap. It is important to wash your neck, as it also requires much care. With the recipes below you will have moist and smooth skin.

Recipe 1

In a cup pour 3 tablespoons of honey, half of green lemon juice then prepare the mixture, apply it to your face and neck for 15 minutes. Remove the mask with a generous amount of warm water.

Recipe 2

In a mixing bowl put three tablespoons of facial clay and a tablespoon and a half of honey, mix then apply to your face and neck leaving it to sit for twenty minutes and then immediately rinse with plenty of warm water.

Recipe 3

Two tablespoons of honey then add an egg yolk then mix perfectly until you reach a creamy consistency.

Apply this mixture on your face and neck and leave it on for a period of 20 minutes then remove the mask with plenty of warm water.

For Oily Skin and Acne Problems

The following masks will help you solve your skin's Sebaceous overproduction, as well as to improve acne problems.

Recipe 1

Whisk an egg up to a creamy consistency and add lemon juice and half a tablespoon of brown sugar, cover your face and neck with this mixture and let it sit for a period of twenty-five minutes, finally rinse with fresh water.

Recipe 2

In a blender add half of a cucumber, a quarter of a red apple and an egg-white, then blend until you reach a paste consistency.

Apply the mixture to your face and neck and let it sit for twenty-five minutes and immediately remove it with by washing your face with plenty of warm water.

Recipe 3

In a bowl place a boiled potato and using a fork, crush to a paste then add two tablespoons of milk and half of a lemons juice. Apply on your face and neck and let it act for a period of twenty minutes and removed with plenty of warm water.

. . . .

For Mixed Skin

. . . .

It's surprising that many people have mixed skin but with this simple recipe it can be easily extracted from *my most intimate secrets and* will help eliminate the problem and as a result produce a spectacularly normal skin.

Recipe 1

In a bowl add zest from one lemon, two tablespoons of powdered milk, a spoonful of barley and gradually add warm water to make a paste. Using your fingertips apply paste to your face and neck in a circular motion while massaging your face to stimulate the circulation for a period of one minute and a half. Let it sit for thirty minutes then wash away with plenty of fresh water.

It's a great secret that helps the skin stay fresh and young for many years.

Another one of my big secrets that is fabulous is this simple mask that gives amazing results after the first application. Red wine contains high levels of antioxidants, which helps in a magical way to regenerate smooth and youthful skin especially when combined with honey:

Recipe 2

Mix two tablespoons of red wine with four tablespoons of honey. Apply to your face and neck leaving it to act for twenty-five minutes. Rinse your face with plenty of ice water. From the beginning of your application, you will experience an unparalleled sensation.

Another fabulous secret that has been saved with great zeal by major entertainment figures for their immediate results at the time of application will help keep skin youthful and hydrated;

also minimizes fine lines, dark circles, blemishes caused by age and acts as an anti-inflammatory remedy. It's mentioned below:

Recipe 3

You will need: 4 slices of bread without the crust, 1 cup of cold whole milk, 4 tablespoons of instant oats, twenty drops of l lime juice and 2 slices of potato or cucumber (whatever you have).

Procedure:

Using a flat plate, spread the four slices of bread to form an envelope size sheet and using a spoon spread the whole milk over the bread evenly and with the same spoon crushed the slices of bread so they join each other.

Then take Instant Oatmeal flakes and spread them on the mashed up bread, finally add the droplets of lemon over this preparation. Next apply it to your face and neck to form a mask, leaving free the area of the eyes and the nostrils.

Place sliced cucumber or potato over your eyes. Take a little time to unwind for approximately twenty minutes, then remove the mask with your hands and finally rinse with plenty of cold water.

This mask is very effective and you can use it at least once a month. It is also highly recommended to use it before an event, since your appearance will look fresh and radiant.

You can also apply it after a big event, to recover from the hustle and bustle of the night before. I am sure that you will love this mask.

Enjoy the results!

CHAPTER 4

The Importance of Eyebrow and Eyelash Care

For both men and women the care and attention of eyebrows and eyelashes is very important. Eyebrows and hair form the contours of the face. Eyebrows are the frame of the eyes and their form creates expressions that will make you look happy, sad, angry or tired.

In extreme cases, it seems that our eyes are very close together or far apart, giving the appearance of having vision problems. I recommend visiting a professional eyebrow designer so that you can receive help in making a good decision on giving them the correct shape.

To preserve your eyebrow appearance, continue visiting a professional eyebrow designer once every month and a half.

To strengthen your eyebrows and eyelashes, I would like to recommend the following:

Recipe 1

In a small jar, mix equal parts of the following oils: Castor oil, sweet almond oil and avocado oil.

Every night, take a drop of the oil mix and using your index finger and thumb, rub together and warm the oil between your fingers.

Continue to massage each eyebrow back forward with the oil and vice versa to the other eyebrow for thirty seconds. Next take another drop and warm it up using your fingers to now give a gentle massage to your lashes.

This treatment will help strengthen your eyebrows and eyelashes and look more abundant.

You can also add five drops of this oil mixture to your mascara or clay mask since the properties of these three oils benefit greatly to your eyelashes in each application.

Recipe 2(to drink)

An excellent preparation consists of: carrot juice from 2 carrots, orange juice from four oranges, one tablespoon of honey, a tablespoon of walnut, a tablespoon of pine nuts, a tablespoon of pollen from flowers.

This recipe produces a juice with the mentioned ingredients that can be taken in the mornings for a length of a month and a half. Your lashes will be stronger and more beautiful as a result of the vitamins that you will have added to this juice.

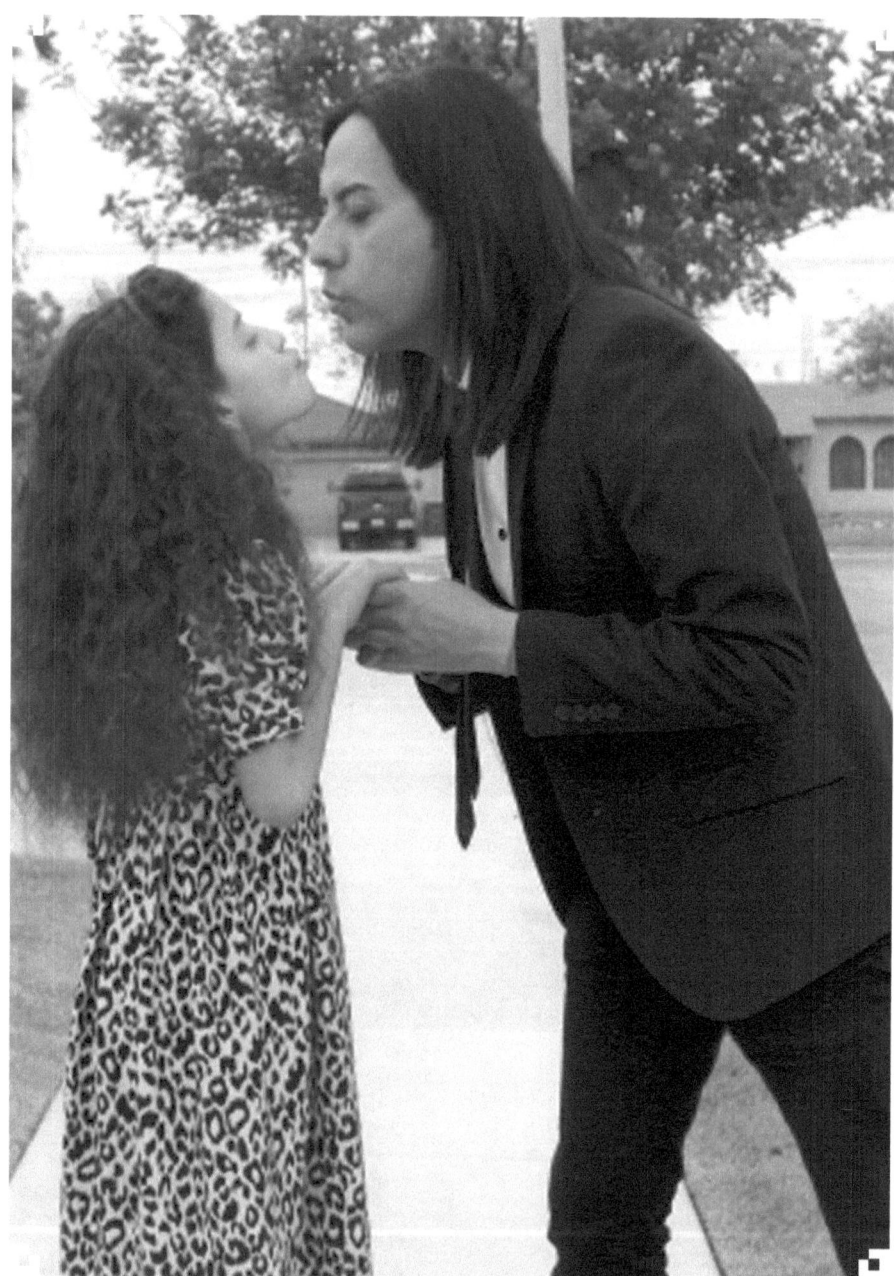

CHAPTER 5

The Magic of Having and Maintaining Enviable Lips

I find it difficult to understand why the majority of people have forgotten this essential part of their face.

It is of utmost importance to provide attention and care of aesthetics to our lips, as to any other part of our body, since they are also affected directly by different climate changes, the rays of the Sun, the air, cold and age.

The alternatives offered by the cosmetic companies are usually commercial lipsticks, which usually contain chemicals and dyes that are far from benefiting your lips, often damaging, diminishing natural color, while making lips dry and sensitive.

So let me give you some remedies that will solve these problems and help you have healthy, beautiful and luscious lips.

Recipe 1

Chocolate lip balm

For its preparation you'll need a quarter teaspoon of grated chocolate, a teaspoon of cocoa butter, a teaspoon of coconut oil and a teaspoon of vitamin "E".

Use in a container that you can place into your microwave, place all the ingredients into your container and heat for 30 seconds. Stir until blended. Wait until it has cooled and apply it on your lips and also before you use your lipstick.

Recipe 2

Lip balm.

For this you will need 2 tablespoons of calendula oil, half a tablespoon of grated beeswax, 2 tablespoons of cocoa butter and oil of wheat.

Melt all your ingredients over a stove in a saucepan until blended. Pour the melted ingredients into small glass jars and store them so that they may be kept in good condition. Once cooled, apply to chapped lips.

Recipe 3

Lip gloss

This lip gloss is excellent to use on top of your lipstick that will give you a wet and sexy look. You can also use it as a balm on natural lips. The ingredients are: 1 teaspoon of honey and 3 teaspoons of cocoa butter.

To prepare, melt these ingredients over a stove in a sauce pan. Pour the melted ingredients into glass containers and start enjoying the benefits.

CHAPTER 6

Dentral Care

. . . .

Smile Care

. . . .

To have a sexy smile and maintain not only healthy teeth, but your own health, there are infallible rules that we have to meet. First off visit your dentist twice a year and your Dentist recommendations should be followed to the 'T'.

As a tip, I recommend to make your first visit days before your birthday to have it as a reference for an important date and also to consider it six months later for the next visit.

The fact that you brush your teeth in a vigorous manner is not sufficient nor does it mean that your gums and teeth will be completely clean, but rather the only thing you will achieve is damaging the enamel and your gums. I suggest you use a medium bristle brush and you brush at a forty-five degree angle in a circular motion for a period of not less than three minutes.

If at all possible avoid drinks such as tea, as well as others that contain caffeine, red wine, and especially cigarettes, all of these things can stain your teeth gradually.

In the event that you can't help it, try brushing your teeth immediately after you have consumed these drinks or have smoked. That way you help to reduce unpleasant stains.

I also recommend that you avoid from eating too often, any foods and beverages containing citrus, because they degrade the enamel of your teeth due to the acids. With citrus, your teeth lose their protective minerals, you have to give them time to recover and if you brush them you will very easily remove a layer of enamel, which is not recommendable.

Tip:

To keep teeth white with a homemade recipe, moisten your brush with a mixture of baking soda and water, add the toothpaste of your choice and then brush in the usual way.

This homemade recipe is to be used only one time per week or otherwise you could make your teeth and gums too sensitive.

Mouthwashes will be your best allies, since they will not only help you after you brush your teeth but ensure a thorough cleaning and prolong a pleasant breath.

They can be used as an alternative, albeit in a sporadic manner, when you don't have the opportunity to brush your teeth as you should normally.

Flossing should be unconditional because it will help keep your gums and teeth healthy.

Pastes that contain bleach will require special attention, because they contain abrasives that precisely help to achieve whiter teeth. However, don't abuse them because you want to avoid future sensitivity problems. Don't forget to brush three times a day.

And remember: There is nothing that can compare to a beautiful smile!

CHAPTER 7

The Secrets to Makeup

Without a doubt our face is what draws the most attention to our bodies. For this reason a great time should be spent at minimum to study our facial features and discover our strengths and weaknesses.

In all accounts with large eyes you will need to find a way to disguise them and draw little attention to them however, if your eyes are very tiny and separated, you must learn to make them appear normal to cause the opposite effect.

Although there are many different types of eyes and looks, some general rules will facilitate the tasks and diagnosis.

. . . .
TYPE OF EYES
. . . .

Wide-set eyes: The nose as a halfway point, allows you to realize that the eyes are separated because they are basically away from the nose.

Sunken eyes: Easily detectable by its appearance, with a sense of looking sad and sagging, by this you must pay greater attention to the colors of makeup you can apply to make them appear happier.

Big eyes: They transmit confidence and security however, you must make sure the colors of makeup you apply features there beauty.

Small eyes: Without a doubt the most common, but they also have their own charm and if you apply perfect makeup techniques you will get the desired effect.

BRUSHES AND APPLICATORS FOR EYE MAKEUP

It is necessary that you purchase brushes, utensils, and shadows, adequate and of good quality to avoid damaging your skin.

Thick brushes: This will help you when using shadows in powder form in different colors.

Elongated, short-bristled brushes: Helps when applying color to blend the shadow in the crease of the eyelids. They are very useful for light colors with dark tints. Its major use is in the wide areas of the eyelid, near the eyebrow which is the brow bone.

Brushes with sponges: The sponge absorbs the color so that it can extend in larger quantities. They are highly recommended when applying dark colors, as they deepen color and it gives more shape to the eye.

Mascara for the eyelashes: The black is commonly used to give a natural appearance to our lashes and can be used on any color of lashes.

Eyelash Curler: This is a bit of basic use for those people who have extremely limp eyelashes and have had them since birth. When using an eyelash curler, apply gentle pressure to avoid damaging and breaking of lashes.

MY TREASURED AND MOST INTIMATE SECRETS

My treasured and most intimate secrets about makeup, I place these at your fingertips and make available so that you can achieve a new image worthy of a Hollywood diva!

Skin preparation

To achieve perfect makeup, skin must be prepared prior to get that soft peach skin appearance.

Step number one.

Begin by washing your face with a mild soap to ensure your skin is clean and free of impurities. Apply a moisturizer according to your skin type. Then take some ice cubes and wrap them in a wash cloth and then rub your face and neck with the washcloth, this ensures a perfect moisturizer. It will help seal the moisturizer and close your pores to prolong the life of your makeup.

Step number two.

How to choose a perfect makeup base? Your arm and forearm are two completely different skin tones, obviously one is light and the other one is dark. Test a makeup base and apply a couple of drops on your arm and then on your forearm, taking into consideration that the base will be a tone lighter than the color of your skin.

Initially you will notice that the color looks clear, but after a few minutes, you will notice how it adapts to your skin tone, giving you a perfect appearance.

. . . .

SKIN CORRECTORS
CORRECTION OF IMPERFECTIONS AND POWDERS

. . . .

Concealers

Concealers can be used as a form of correction to imperfections and come in the form of a lipstick and has a creamy base. Always use a shade lighter than the natural color of your skin. Use concealer on dark circles and dark spots.

The perfect way to apply is by drawing a straight line under your eyes. Then using the tip of your middle finger, blend the corrector softly to distribute evenly. You will be your own judge to determine where you must use it to cover the dark spots or dark circles without blending away the corrector.

Translucent powder

This product is a very important weapon, since its function is to cover the beautiful superficial surface of the skin, to avoid an oily appearance and above all to extend the life of your makeup. The application will be with the help of a special powder thick round brush.

Apply the powder in a circular motion covering the face, neck and don't be afraid to pass it over eyelids and lips since this will serve as a base for the application of shadows, mascaras and lipsticks.

. . . .

Eyebrow shaping with powder

. . . .

Using an angle brush and a shadow color as close to the natural tone of your eyebrows, find the natural shape to draw their outline while highlighting their natural beauty.

The eye shadows

A sure way to make your eyes pop is to use neutral colors such as: beige, brown, gray, white and black, because they are easy to match with any color of clothing and they are perfect for any skin tone.

The light and soft colors must be used on areas where the light is reflected to create a shade of color, continuing with medium color tones, these must be applied on the eyelid, then use eyeliner pencils in black or charcoal and gently trace a line following the natural shape of the top and bottom of your lashes.

It ends with the application of mascara. Remember that your application is from root to tips. You will have to repeat it as many times necessary to acquire thickness and the desired length, getting sexy and beautiful effect that you are looking for but avoid clumps.

I highly recommend this application of makeup for all types of eye shapes, primarily for small eyes, the effect of light is greatly pronounced by these colors.

Makeup for large to medium-sized eyes: I suggest using soft tones on the areas in which they reflect more light to create an artificial shade. Then it gives a touch of a lighter shadow under the brow and on the eyelid. Use colors that match the color tone of clothing that you've chosen to wear for the day.

Finally, I suggest you use an eye liner especially on top of the eyelids. The line thickness will depend on how much you want to minimize their appearance. With respect to the bottom line of the eye, I recommend to follow the natural line to make your lashes look great.

For people who have bulging eyes, never wear eye shadows with shimmers or light colors. It is better that you avoid them as much as possible. Matte tones are the most suitable for these eye shapes, this way you can correct and improve their appearance.

BLUSH APPLICATION

This depends on the type of makeup you choose to wear.

I'll give you some tips that will give you a harmonious and natural look that will highlight your beauty.

The blush application usually goes on prior to applying lipstick and immediately after eye shadow. Although this is not a general rule, so if you want, you can apply it at the end of your make up to balance the colors.

The perfect blush color is the natural color of your rosy cheeks, so by pinching your cheeks a little by using your fingers, the color that results from this action will show you your natural color and you should try to match it with a blush.

Remember that your blush will be a complement to your skin, not to your lipstick; one of the most common mistakes women make is the use of a blush that matches their lipstick with an end result of being either too pale or too dark.

Different blush tones are usually used to draw attention to certain points and to sculpt the face, but to do this we need to be very skilled and is regularly used for night makeup more than daily day makeup.

You will notice that blush comes in several different presentations from liquid, cream and powder. It is here where I share with you another of my professional makeup secrets: Regularly, I prefer the powder blush to give a very natural touch that can't be in any way compared to other blush forms. Only in cases of very dry skin will I only use blush in cream or liquid form because they give you a touch of hydration.

For the application it is essential to make use of a professional brush if you want a better finish. In the market there are two types of brushes, the angle and the normal round shape.

The brush size should be in proportion to the size of your face. Load your brush with the blush of your choice and then shake it to remove excess powder. For a better guideline, smile big then apply blush to your cheeks while applying with rotating movements, stop smiling and then extend the color with your brush towards your temples or ears, without actually applying them to the temples or ears of course, and this is done in a brushing manner that you can repeat in case the blush is not distributed enough. The liquid blush should be applied with a sponge or your fingertips.

In case your face is round or wide apply blush at the tip of the cheekbone trying to keep it in the area below the area of the eye otherwise, if you extend the blush color, your face will look wider. The darker blush colors should be used only in cases of dramatic makeup and for party nights.

There is another type of blush called a bronzer that is strictly for the summer season since they basically reflect exposure to the sun. Bronzers come in shades of orange and up to a roasted coffee color. This helps your skin give off the appearance of a good summer vacation.

. . . .

How to Choose the Right Lip Color

. . . .

CHOOSING THE RIGHT LIP COLOR FOR YOUR LIPS

There is a wide variety of lip colors, although there is only one way of applying. I suggest that when you go to buy it, be sure that the lipstick contains moisturizers.

When applying lipstick, it is necessary to begin by outlining them with a neutral lip liner pencil along the natural lines of your lips. Also you can apply to the outer edges of your lips lightly only if you have very thin lips using a lip brush. Fill in the rest of your lips with lipstick in an easy way and finally you can use a napkin by blotting it in between your lips, to remove the excess and to seal your lipstick.

In this application, I ask for special attention to the following rule: The amount of makeup applied to your face, should be related to the hours of the day; for example: during the early hours of the morning, when you have a greater amount of natural light, use less amounts of makeup, as well as less depth of it. During the evening you should use more makeup and contouring due to the absence of natural light.

Use your common sense by following this simple rule and you will have a spectacular appearance, makeup that is worthy of any diva!

CHPATER 8

Bust Care

. . . .

STRATEGIES TO MAINTAIN A FIRM
AND YOUTHFUL BUST

. . . .

The bust is a part of the body that most women don't provide proper care, while bringing on problems ranging from stretch marks to sagging caused by age, up and down with weight, bad habits, pregnancy and lactation. Let me then offer you a list of ideas to follow so that you keep a firm, beautiful and youthful bust.

Tip number one

I recommend maintaining a stable diet and when you want to decrease it, it has to be gradual, not sudden, uncontrolled weight loss can bring a consequence of making your bust flaccid.

Tip number two

Good posture is really important. Look at yourself in the mirror all around and correct your posture by standing up straight, this will balance your body and make your breasts look lifted.

Tip number three

Make sure that the type of BRA you buy is suitable for the size of your bust.

If you used a bra one size less than yours, it will cause you discomfort and marks and if you wear a bra one size bigger than your size, you still won't get the desired needed support.

Tip number four

The exercise that helps the upper part of the torso and arms are wonderful to keep the firmness of your breasts.

Tip number five

Take a small rubber ball and with your arms extended forward, try to tighten by squeezing with some force for ten seconds, repeating this exercise at least five times a day.

Tip number six

Using the palms of your hands, bring them closer to your chest like you're going to pray and press them together for a few seconds, repeat it at least five times a day.

One last very effective Tip:

Lye on the floor, take a one pound weight in each hand or bottles of water, hold them with your hands up vertically without bending the elbows ten times in a row once a day.

A very special recommendation: Examine your breasts regularly to identify any changes by doing the following: place one arm behind your head and support your head then with the other hand using your fingers, touch around the breast and in or around your armpits, repeat the same action on the other side, one or two days after your period.

If you detect any lump, abnormality or sensitivity, consult your Gynecologist immediately.

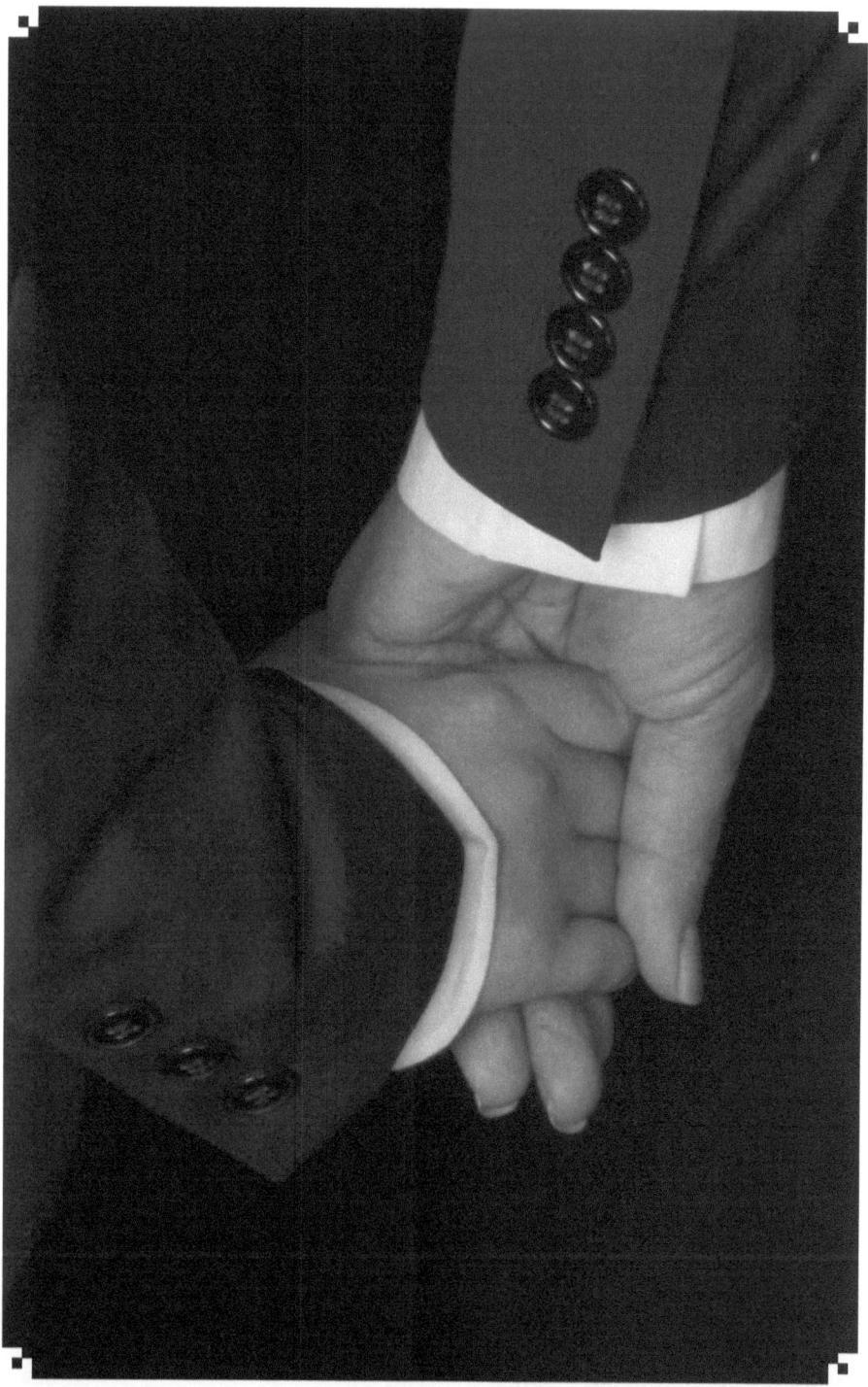

CHAPTER 9

Feet and Hand Care

HAND CARE

. . . .

Hands are an important part of the body which certainly reveals something about our personality. However, due to our day-to-day activities, we use them and expose them to attacks of every moment by the use of products such as detergents, cleaners, chlorine, cold, heat and water.

So, it is of the utmost importance to provide extraordinary care by subjecting them to different treatments of hydration and nutrition to be able to have soft hands with a nice appearance.

There are a number of home treatments that I will indicate for you that are applied at the spas where celebrities go. These will enhance the beauty of those special parts of your personality which are your hands which forms that part of you.

Treatment number one

In a bowl just fill it halfway with warm water then place one tablespoon of wheat germ and five drops of lemon zest. Mix all these ingredients and dip your hands until the water passes from warm to cold. Take your hands and grab a little sugar, using your fingers spread it all over your hands.

Rub both your hands together while giving yourself a massage. Sugar is a natural exfoliator that helps to get rid of dead skin cells so that your skin feels and looks more refined.

In addition, the discoloration of your skin will be approximately two shades lighter from its usual color.

Finally dry your hands and add a natural moisturizer that you will prepare based on five drops of Glycerin and five drops of rose water. Rub your hands until this lotion is gone. The feeling will leave you speechless!

Treatment number two

This procedure has to be practiced at night before you go to sleep.

Prepared from honey and a boiled potato - peel the boiled potato to get a smooth consistency. Then place it in a bowl and add three tablespoons of honey and a splash of milk. Beat all these ingredients together. Then apply this paste and massage your hands for five minutes.

Then rest your hands for 15 minutes, then rinse with enough running water, continue drying your hands gently. Now take a few drops of olive oil and give yourself a massage with these drops. Then put on a pair of cotton gloves and go to bed. Remove the gloves the next morning.

Treatment number three

Home treatment with whole milk in the evening before you go to sleep

Place some whole milk in a bowl halfway with half a cup of lemon juice. Dip your hands in these ingredients for ten minutes and end by rinsing your hands with warm water. Then add six drops of Glycerin in the palm of your hands and give yourself a gentle massage until the greasy feeling disappears. The results are impressive.

How to Have Healthy, Strong and Clear Nails

Nails reveal a big part of your personality; similar to your hands, they constitute the better part of you. Remember that the little things count.

Here are some small, but very important details to keep the good health and appearance of your nails.

By no means should you ever bite your nails to the cuticles. To prevent against the harsh damage from detergents, soaps, and other cleaning supplies that you may use in different household cleaning chores, use rubber gloves. These help to avoid the contact with these harmful ingredients to maintain the health of your nails and hands.

Lastly, trim your nails after you come out of the shower.

My recommendation:

It is best to file your nails with care and proportionally to an aesthetic form, for the most part, avoid cutting them with small scissors or nail clippers. Paint your nails with polishes of good quality avoiding the fast-dry enamels because they are made with an acetone base ingredient that is highly damaging which causes discoloration and brittleness.

Stay away from nail polish removers with an acetone base and choose solvent-free nail polish removers.

Avoid at all costs the mania of biting your nails. The first thing that you have

to do is to overcome stress, anxiety, and above all shyness. Seek the help of your Physician to prescribe vitamins such as these: vitamin B1, vitamin B2 and Vitamin D.

Recipe 1

Also use polishes with aloe, this will help make your nails stronger and give you such an unpleasant taste if you ever try to bite your nails again.

Recipe 2

Grab a cotton ball and soak it in white vinegar and rub your nails with it. This technique will give you the natural whiteness with guaranteed results.

Recipe 3

Make a mixture of baking soda with water and then use a soft small brush and grab the mixture with the brush and brush underneath your nails.

Recipe 4

Try and practice this effective recipe for at least once a month to clarify and remove stains from your nails. Soak your nails in 250 ml of hot water and add a tablespoon of hydrogen peroxide for ten minutes.

Recipe 5

A simple recipe to help improve the strength of your nails and cuticles, would be to rub a cotton soaked in olive oil and a few drops of vitamin B.

Recipe 6

For fragile nails there is nothing better than to leave them soaked in a mixture of mineral water and seaweed powder, both are rich in Silicone. Prepare this mixture and soak your nails for twenty minutes and repeat this treatment at least four times a month until you see healthy and strong nails.

Care of the feet

How could we forget the most important part of our body? Foot care is essential. Also don't forget the support they have given us throughout our lives, from our first steps until this day to perform our daily activities, enjoying a good walk by the beach or the park and why not? Even... dancing!

A host of things that I could mention without a doubt for those who do care is our weight and the different paths we've taken. There are more than enough reasons to provide the utmost care to thank our feet for all that they do for us.

Unfortunately, age, disease, poor circulation, the use of wrong shoe sizes that are not for us, poorly cut nails, etc., have negative effects on our feet. Certain problems tend to be, certainly, some symptoms serious medical conditions: such as arthritis, diabetes or neurological disorders and blood circulation.

To prevent these problems, we should treat them very well paying close attention to your feet on a regular basis with the help of a Podiatrist. This physician specializes in providing special treatment appropriately although in most cases, you may need to resort to an orthopedist or with a dermatologist for skin problems.

Routine 1

After your daily activities, including your job, sit or lie down and elevate your feet at a height of two feet or approximately sixty centimeters. Once they're up, perform some stretching exercises and circular movements gently for 10 minutes, especially if you were sitting or standing for long periods of time.

Routine 2

In a small tub where you can submerge your feet, add some warm water, 4 tablespoons of Epsom salt and a cup of hot milk. Relax your feet in this water for twenty minutes. Towel dry your feet then continue with the help of a hair dryer, blow dry your feet until they have been completely dry between the toes and nails.

This is a great time to give yourself a gentle massage with good oil, preferably that of sweet almond, since it will help to stimulate circulation to your feet.

Routine 3

Use a pumice stone when you shower, gently rubbing around the heels this will help you to avoid and eliminate hardening skin. Finish drying your feet as suggested before and add a few drops of Glycerin to provide more softness.

Routine 4

At least once a month before you go to sleep, massage your feet with cocoa butter, then cover them with a plastic bag and put on some socks. The next morning you will have soft, silky feet.

If you have tired and sore feet, soak them in a tub of warm water with 5 drops of lavender essential oil and 2 tablespoons of sea salt, for about 25 minutes.

Sea salt is an excellent way to soothe pain to your feet when used with the combination of warm water, which is also beneficial for preventing infections of the skin, pain, or cracks.

For the most part, the lavender oil has healing powers that are essential to relieve the pain of muscles while leaving a rich nice smell to your feet.

Remember that after each bath, it is an ideal time to file your nails.

CHAPTER 10

Care of Elbows and Knees

Elbows and knees are very easily to treat body parts but are too often forgotten.

There are four basic methods of body and facial beauty. Cleaning, nutrition, exfoliation and hydration, has to be done to your whole body however, I am sure that we don't pay a lot of attention to these treatments and how to apply them correctly to those parts where they are much needed.

Certainly without a doubt the overlying skin around the elbows and knees are the most rough and dry parts of the body. Just imagine how the top skin suffers from lack of care and attention, causing them to become very rough looking and unattractive.

These parts are extremely exposed and their sebaceous glands are unevenly distributed, coupled with the friction of our clothing and objects that further worsen their appearance. I assure you that you won't have beautiful legs and sexy arms without giving yourself the appropriate care to your elbows and knees.

Recipe 1

Take a warm bath to soften your skin. Prep some butter, fine sea salt and almond oil. Mix these ingredients to a creamy consistency to give yourself a massage in circular motions for 5 minutes on each knee and elbow. Next, remove with warm water and then end by applying some almond oil to your knees and elbows.

Recipe 2

Another effective recipe is as follows: mix two teaspoons of sugar and the same amount of lemon juice then give yourself a gentle massage for approximately 2 to 4 minutes, leaving it on for several minutes then rinse.

Recipe 3

Lemon can be used by itself. Squeeze a lemon and soak it up with a cotton ball and then rub it on these parts of your body.

Important note: you must never expose yourself to the Sun after applying lemon juice, since the results will revert to making your skin much darker.

Recipe 4

Another very effective option and this will give you excellent results, is to apply some yogurt mixed with oats. Apply the yogurt mix and let it sit for ten minutes then, lightly rinse and dry your skin leaving it slightly damp to take advantage of this hydration recipe.

Recipe 5

Make a combination with half a lemon juice or aloe vera, 2 tablespoons of brown sugar, a tablespoon of olive oil and some drops of essence of jasmine. After you've bathed, apply the mixture with either a Luffa or a sponge. Rub this paste on the affected areas for approximately five minutes. Continue by rinsing yourself slightly and allow your skin to absorb the benefits.

All these treatments should be performed at least once a week until you notice results. Then, as maintenance, apply them once a month.

CHAPTER 11

Prevention and Treatment of Stretch Marks

The relaxation of the skin is the main cause of the breakdown of the elasticity thus causing us to have stretch marks.

Particularly affected areas are: the upper arm, belly, thighs chest and buttocks. When stretch marks appear they are very easy to identify, as they begin in a blueish-red color and later change to a red to a yellowish-white.

I must let you know that this problem was previously believed to affect only females.

This begins to appear in adolescents, without distinction of sex, although in the case of men, body hair tends to be beneficial because it makes stretch marks go unnoticed.

The factors that lead to this condition are: the stretching of the skin by pregnancy, sudden changes in connective tissue volume which serves to unite and give structure to the different parts of the body and up to constipation; some hormonal irregularities weaken general tissues and at the same time prevent the formation of the cells of the fibroblasts in the dermis and epidermis.

Finally, having nervous system problems can alter the respiration and the oxygen if irregular, altering the condition of the skin.

Solution

Reactivate the damaged tissues by doing it the following way: take some sweet almond oil and use your thumb and index rubbing the oil between the fingers and pinch the stretch mark with gentle movement and roll the skin with those two fingers at the same time; repeat ten times in a row, every two days.

A great ally to improve the appearance of stretch marks is exercise because it activates the blood circulation and improves the elasticity of your skin.

In the case of pregnant women, it is very important to have hydration of the skin at the abdomen so the elastic fibers are tightened without breaking due to the increase in volume. In this case, give yourself a soft massage to the abdomen making use of sweet almond oil. This massage should be performed daily after shower and throughout the pregnancy.

CHAPTER 12

Tips and Tricks for Cellulite

Cellulite is not anything other than the accumulation of a jelly-like matter that is composed of water, fat and toxins below the subcutaneous tissue.

People who lead a sedentary lifestyle, which is exceeded in the food by ingestion of toxic substances to the body, a poor ovarian function, emotional changes, and decompensation of the **neurovegetative** system, are some of the elements that favor this condition.

Both sex's indiscriminately deal with the condition, although definitely women are the ones who frequently suffer from cellulite.

The strategic points where we can observe this training are: The abdomen, hips, back, spine, lower part very common on the outer side of the arms and the neck. Although with regularity it can be confused with obesity, especially in the knees and ankles which is even more noticeable in the external surface of the thighs.

The war against cellulite must be steady and never let your guard down. There are several treatments for prevention and I will reveal some of my best secrets:

❖ First of all lead a very healthy, active life avoiding sitting or standing for long periods. Exercising, cycling, yoga and water sports are particularly extraordinary in helping you in the process.

❖ With regards to food, stay away from large amounts of salt, red meat, fatty seafood, chocolate and spices. Drinking water is a must outside of just eating meals.

❖ Circulation is very important for a healing treatment. I recommend you give yourself a dry massage to your entire body in the privacy of your bathroom with a friction mitt, making constant circular movements medium pressure, for ten minutes. Then moisten with warm water and natural soap with a friction mitt and again repeat the massages for another ten minutes. Give yourself a massage with a friction hose and some cold water to firm your tissues.

CHAPTER 13

My Ten Most Intimate Secrets

(Never Revealed)

"These are my ten largest and intimate secrets never revealed"

"Today I want to share them with you so that, like many of the famous you may enjoy the amazing benefits that I've been the first to experience.

These secrets have been obtained through many years of research, experiences and above all personal practice to make the dramatic results I have proven."

. . . .
Secret Number One
. . . .

Rejuvenation prepared with fruits of the forest.

This preparation will help keep you young, full of energy and with a spectacular looking skin due to the antioxidant properties of these fruits that have been tested at a scientific level, particularly its benefits to rejuvenate.

In a food processor, place half a glass of water and ten of each of these fruits: strawberries, blackberries, raspberries and blueberries. All these fruits are seasonal, and in case you can't find any of them, then don't worry just use whatever is at your fingertips. Next, add two tablespoons of honey and blend to make sure that they thoroughly have been combined then pour it into a glass and drink it.

Make sure that the fruit is fresh, completely clean and disinfected. Get accustomed to drinking this smoothie at least twice a week in the morning as your breakfast.

. . . .

Secret Number Two

. . . .

A different drink

Choose a Jell-O of the flavor of your choice. In an eight-ounce bottle of natural water, add the full package, cover and shake until it dissolves completely. Now you have a refreshing drink that you can take all day or at any time to quench your thirst, without the pretext that you don't like natural water; so hydrate your body and you'll get the vitamins needed for your hair and nails.

The gelatin is not anything other than keratin. Keratin is a substance which is an integral part of the outer layers of the epidermis and some of the organs that are derived from are: the hair, the nails and the skin. Take advantage of the benefits this drink will give you.

The recipe is simple and easy with extraordinary results that you can see and feel.

I recommend drinking this as you would as often as water. It is very good for everyone, especially those having hair problems like thinning and also brittle nails. As a special note, it acquires packets of sugar-free Jell-O to avoid the calories and the weight gain.

. . . .

Secret Number Three

. . . .

Preparation of Rosewater and Glycerin

This mixture is ideal after your bath. The benefits are wonderful and it helps keep your skin free of impurities. For this recipe, it will be almost difficult to ever get outbreaks like pimples and blackheads if you suffer from it. To achieve a skin tone that looks firmer you can use it on all parts of your body, including the face.

To develop this rosewater and Glycerin, you will need: six ounces of ethyl alcohol, the petals of four red roses, two ounces of liquid Glycerin and a 16 oz. glass bottle.

Once you've gathered all these ingredients, begin by placing the rose petals into the bottle and pouring the liquid Glycerin and finally incorporate the ethyl alcohol into the bottle. Cap the bottle and shake this mixture. Let it sit for ten days in a cool place with low light.

You can start using this mixture once the ten days are up. Remember to apply it on all parts of your body rubbing the solution with your hands.

It is highly recommended to be applied as a toner after cleansing and moisturizing your face and neck. Apply it gently by using a cotton ball.

. . . .
Secret Number Four
. . . .

Care of the neck

It is amazing to see how the vast majority of people take care of their entire body, daily cleaning, moisturizing, hydrating and toning, but overlooking this part of your body: the neck, just like any other body part also suffers from mistreatment, inclement weather, the law of gravity and above all that unavoidable factor which is time.

So there is no reason you should forget to give your neck the proper care that it also deserves. So follow the same routine you would do at the time of your daily facial care by applying the same products to your neck.

Add an exercise routine that you'll do in the morning and at night.

Begin by standing in a straight posture and turn your face from side to side doing it slowly, ensuring that your chin touches your shoulder repeating this exercise 20 times, then with your head looking straight move your head up and down another 20 times, moving your head as far back and as far down as possible.

This routine ensures that the skin around your neck stays toned, youthful and will also provide you with relaxation.

· ·

Secret Number Five

· ·

The lemon

The lemon is a fruit with great clarifying properties that contains Vitamin C, low in sugars, potassium and sodium, which is used in different weight loss regimens.

To clear spots, at night add a few drops of Glycerin and lemon juice, rub your skin with this mixture and you'll notice how gradually your skin will take an even tone, clear and free of spots. Be cautious and use this recipe only at night, by day it would cause the opposite effect.

The same recipe can be used when you bathe to treat your back, do it by applying these ingredients to your back using a towel soaked with water as hot as you can stand it and rub that part of your body. The result will be clean and acne free and above all a very smooth back.

As a complement to a weight loss regime, add lemon juice to a half cup of warm water and drink it before eating your food. This will help you reduce fat that causes you to gain weight from carbohydrates and at the same time take a good dose of vitamin C, calorie-free.

For people with problems of high blood pressure it is recommended to replace the salt for lemon in food, because it will serve them as a dressing without the negative effects.

. . . .

Secret Number Six

. . . .

Relaxation and meditation give fabulous results of youth

Relaxation allows you to free yourself from stress, forgetting the everyday problems as well as your plans for the future, because of the level of anxiety that these things may cause.

Meditation, on the other hand, should be directed to thinking positive only.

To begin these routines, prepare your bathtub with water as hot as you can stand it, pour 250 ml. of Lavender oil and incorporate some flowers of your choice.

In your bathroom light seven candles with color and scents of lavender. Both the hot water and lavender oil have relaxing properties that are extraordinary. This combination of aroma and temperature will give you a feeling of relaxation with no other equals.

Lavender oil also causes the same calming effect due to its therapeutic power. Candles give a very special touch and a sense of spiritual serenity to your bathroom.

Finally, play soft instrumental music to create a magical setting. Once you've gathered all these elements, immerse yourself in your tub and treat yourself to forty five minutes of personal love and enjoy the results.

. . . .

Secret Number Seven

. . . .

Facial lifting without scalpel surgery

This secret will give you fabulous results despite being simple you will be totally satisfied; if you practice it often, because its results are cumulative.

It's a mask so effective, that it would be comparable to the idea of taking your face to the gym and exercising it as you do with your body.

Its effect is so notorious that I call it a *facelift surgery without the scalpel*. The ingredients are: 2 egg whites, 10 drops of lemon juice and a teaspoon of rye flour.

In a bowl, put the two egg whites and sprinkle some drops of water. With a fork whisk until it appears to look like snow. Then add a few drops of lemon juice and whisk it a little more so that it can be incorporated into the mix. Then place the bowl in the freezer and let it sit for ten minutes.

Then take out the bowl from the freezer, sprinkle on a teaspoon of rye flour then with a facial brush mix all the ingredients gently.

Now the application is ready for use. Use a hair tie to keep your hair away from your face and apply the mask with a facial brush evenly. Sit back and let the mask sit, now sit in a comfortable position and relax for a forty five minutes.

You'll notice that your skin will slowly begin to dry, feel tense and you will experience the feeling of your muscles working until the end of those incredible forty-five minutes.

Proceed to rinse your face with enough fresh water, until it is free of any residue. As additional information, this mask is perfect for special occasions, since it will leave you ready to enjoy a more youthful face.

. . . .

Secret Number Eight

. . . .

Salmon

The next secret has to do with food, and although previously we have already addressed the issue, this secret has an extraordinary value, that is placed in a special place within *My Ten Biggest Secrets*.

I'm talking about salmon, a fish with great nutritional benefits that could take me several pages to describe, but on this occasion I would like to mention the most interesting benefits.

Among other things it's rich in omega 3 acids and omega 6 which reduces bad cholesterol, plasma triglycerides and reinforces the immune system. In simpler terms, salmon provides nutrients that will give you a good circulation and mind alert.

Without a doubt, your heart will function better and you'll have stronger bones. Your skin will look healthy and fresh, which means that it will keep you youthful for a longer time period.

My recommendation is that you cook it to your liking. Steamed, grilled or in the oven, seasoned with spices of your liking and accompanied with all types of vegetables. You can eat it as often as you wish.

Here's a curious thought? To challenge this fact, take a photograph of yourself before starting a steady intake of salmon as part of your diet for three months then take a new photograph and compare.

Your eyes will not believe the difference.

. . . .

Secret Number Nine

. . . .

The palm of your hand

A golden rule that guarantees a stable weight and good health throughout the years of your life is to practice the rule of consuming food every two hours in portions that would fit in the palm of your hand.

Obviously, it is not to deprive yourself of anything during the day, just simply eating healthier foods often and occasionally giving you small tastes with those maybe-not-so-healthy snacks that you enjoy so much, so eat them as a reward to yourself.

I need to remind you that there are only certain special days (holidays) of the year that you should reward yourself and try to think the same way about these types of food in portions. Pick them cautiously and eat them in moderation.

. . . .

Secret Number Ten

. . . .

Rest and H20

This secret for me is one of the most important to keep you young and healthy. Let's start by talking about the importance of sleep and getting around eight hours of sleep each night or a variation in case that you work on a nightly schedule.

It is essential to understand the importance of rest eight hours daily, if you really want to stay away from wrinkles, dark circles and any physical exhaustion.

Your best weapon will be resting and enjoying your eight hours of sleep. If you are one of those people who have problems sleeping, then you can easily prepare an infusion of herbs, a relaxing tea consisting of infusions from Chamomile, Valerian and lettuce leaves.

These ingredients are easily accessible and are known for their relaxing and tranquil response. Avoid at all cost using any type of sweetener because they will give you an unnecessary burst of energy before your bedtime.

Prepare and drink any of these infusions ten minutes before you go to the bed.

The importance of water

Let us remember that our body constitutes 70% of this element of vital importance to keep the skin moisturized, hydrated and a healthy body. This recommendation could not be missed in my secrets. Sleep quality and water go together hand in hand and are vital elements for many processes of regeneration, cleansing and optimization of functions of our bodies.

Water helps to expel toxins from the food we eat every day and keeps you hydrated. Do not confuse your hunger with thirst.

So drinking water during the day will keep you from overeating and also will help you maintain an ideal weight.

I will mention the right way to use water to achieve its maximum effectiveness in the organism.

- Drink two glasses of water when you wake up in the mornings for this will help to activate your internal organs.

- Drink a glass of water approximately 30 minutes before eating to ensure a better digestion.

- A glass of water before bathing helps to lower blood pressure.

- Something very important to consider and put into practice, is that drinking a glass of water before going to sleep helps your body to prevent strokes and heart attacks.

And so, by doing the two components of this last secret will also contribute to your ability to have a restful sleep.

Choose a book of your liking and get into the habit of reading it ten minutes before you go to sleep.

Dear friends:

In all aspects of life there is always a beginning and an end; up to this point where we are now, I have lived indescribable experiences, full of satisfaction and magic combined in a manner that is special of my secrets and those of the famous to improve health beauty and the culture through My Most Intimate Secrets.

My greatest desire is to place in your hands my knowledge and contribute to your well-being, giving you weapons that allow you to reinvent yourself as being renewed regardless of your age.

Change, improve and practice all my tips to look and feel like a real star in the world of entertainment and the show that is your life itself.

In this book each word, each sentence and each page overflow with all my love, my heart and my soul, contributing to the best of my experiences and knowledge worldwide to whom will have the opportunity to read it.

You can be sure that you will continue to hear news of me. There are still more of my secrets to be revealed.

For now, I invite you to take a brief break, and prepare to discover a new world, a different life and be a person reinvented and renewed with the help of My Most Intimate Secrets and recognizing that the true physical beauty is based on one solid spiritual beauty.

I have the firm conviction that you will very much enjoy putting into practice the content of this work and checking the results themselves.

Best of all is that sometimes when we believe that something is over, it is possible that life continues to surprise us in unexpected ways, so keep your eyes open and continue to explore a little more of My Most Intimate Secrets.

PART II

MY MOST INTIMATE SECRETS

The path to eternal youth

"Exterior beauty does not exist without internal beauty"

Dear friends,

It brings me great joy to reach you through this book, which has been elaborated with all my knowledge, studies and personal experiences lived throughout my life. When I began writing My Most Intimate Secrets, I had very clear details that confirm exterior beauty, especially dieting, which is not only important for living a healthy life but also to reflect radiant beauty throughout your body from the hair on your scalp to the tip of your toes.

However something inside me kept telling me that there is no such thing as exterior beauty without inner beauty. In other words, it doesn't matter how much attention we pay to our exterior if we neglect our most important element, our inner self, our essence and spirit.

My slogan says: *"True beauty begins from within, then out. Begin by feeding your soul, spirit, and every beauty procedure you do will be a complete success."*

I assure you that once you establish contact with your inner self and begin to positively feed it you will be walking directly down the path towards eternal youth.

CHAPTER 14

Life Plan

Everything in life must have an order. It's like counting 1, 2, 3 and progressively so on. It seems simple and logical. Or like going to school, you can't jump from 1st grade to 5th grade there must be a preparation in order to advance in a secure and continuous manner to the next levels.

Most human beings don't make a life plan however those people who have reached success are surely able to trace back their path, planning step by step until reaching their goals and ideals.

For example, let's talk about saving. They say money isn't happiness, but it does bring security and most of all tranquility. Both are very important elements to stay young to avoid uncertainty and mostly stress. This demonstrates how important it is to practice the habit of saving, knowing how to administer your income as well as teaching this to our children.

When I speak of saving I don't only refer to money, I also refer to the better administration of time. Keeping an agenda of daily activities can help you keep track of your time much more efficiently and by doing so you will discover you actually have the time you believed didn't exist for activities you always wanted to accomplish on a regular basis such as; rest and relaxation, meditation or even reading.

In the case of money saving, it is important to do so with a fixed amount according to your income and budget, and keeping it in a safe place where it will increase. Never spend the funds except for a real emergency.

I may be strict with the examples I'm about to provide but there really are certain circumstances that I qualify as emergency situations to justify the spending of the savings fund. Such as being hospitalized for an illness, the passing of a loved one, paying for our children's education and even a well-deserved vacation, this last one may be considered an emergency after a long season of hard work, pressure and stress.

I would like to illustrate this with an example of one of the most successful and wealthiest Women in the world.

Victoria Cecille Moreno

She was born in November 1 1965 in the city of Los Angeles California, where very early she learned the value of family as a priority in life. As a child, she received her first business lessons because Miss Lorena Moreno, mother of Victoria, gave each of her children a savings book along with their usual Sunday allowance, which consists of money for things or food treats, week to week. They managed their income and expenses, checked on their savings book every week. They saw their expenses, purchases and movements and so on, following this rule; the children of Miss Lorena took their own personal balance sheets and developed their own personal finances.

Thereafter, for small Victoria investment and savings became a part of her life. This being her first knowledge about business, would have her obtain her first checkbook, and later buy shares from the Bank of Sweden, while only being 12 years old. The rest is history.

As the years pass and we experience some failures in life, which includes not having any savings. We often think that our life is condemned to continue that way, and at times, we think we are perfect losers.

Let me change your way of thinking to remember that as the day has a beginning and an end, your philosophy could actually be something like this:

"I don't care how many failures I've had in the past, the most important thing now is to plan the success I wish to have tomorrow and in the rest of my future."

Depending on the color with which you paint your world, will be the color in which you live your life.

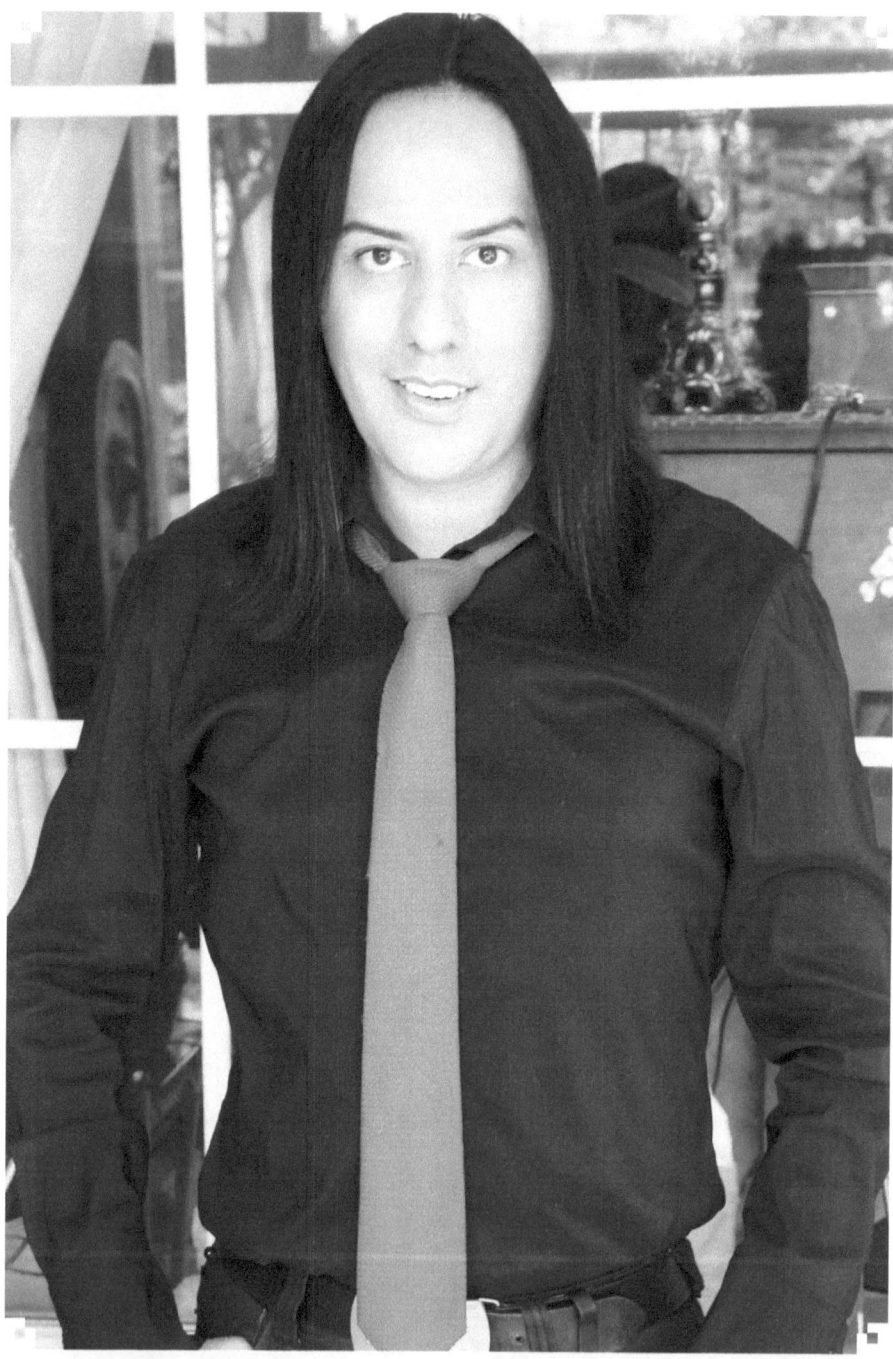

CHAPTER 15

Attitude/Aptitude

· ·
Attitude
· ·

Regardless of how many bad things happen to you, what matters is how you choose to take them, the experiences almost always turn to be positive, if we consider every mistake to be nothing more than a life practice to improve in everything we do.

Practice positive thinking as soon as you open your eyes when you wake up. Program yourself by telling yourself that this day is a beautiful day, full of success, giving the world all the positive energy from you, so that way, you can get the same in return.

· ·
Aptitude
· ·

Aptitude is the ability you have to develop and carry out any activity or task in your daily life.

I invite you to make a personal reconnaissance to find areas where you can perform with greater ease, and become aware of the aspects of your life that are difficult for you. You may develop and carry them out making improvements where required.

Once this analysis is done, it will be much easier for you to put more emphasis on improving all those activities and tasks that hinder you, of course devoting more effort to them to develop the skills needed.

On all those things that are easy, effort and worries will be minor. If any of these areas are difficult for you to work on, remember that in life we all have limitations, but with tenacity, perseverance and commitment you will become a better person, much more complete and happy.

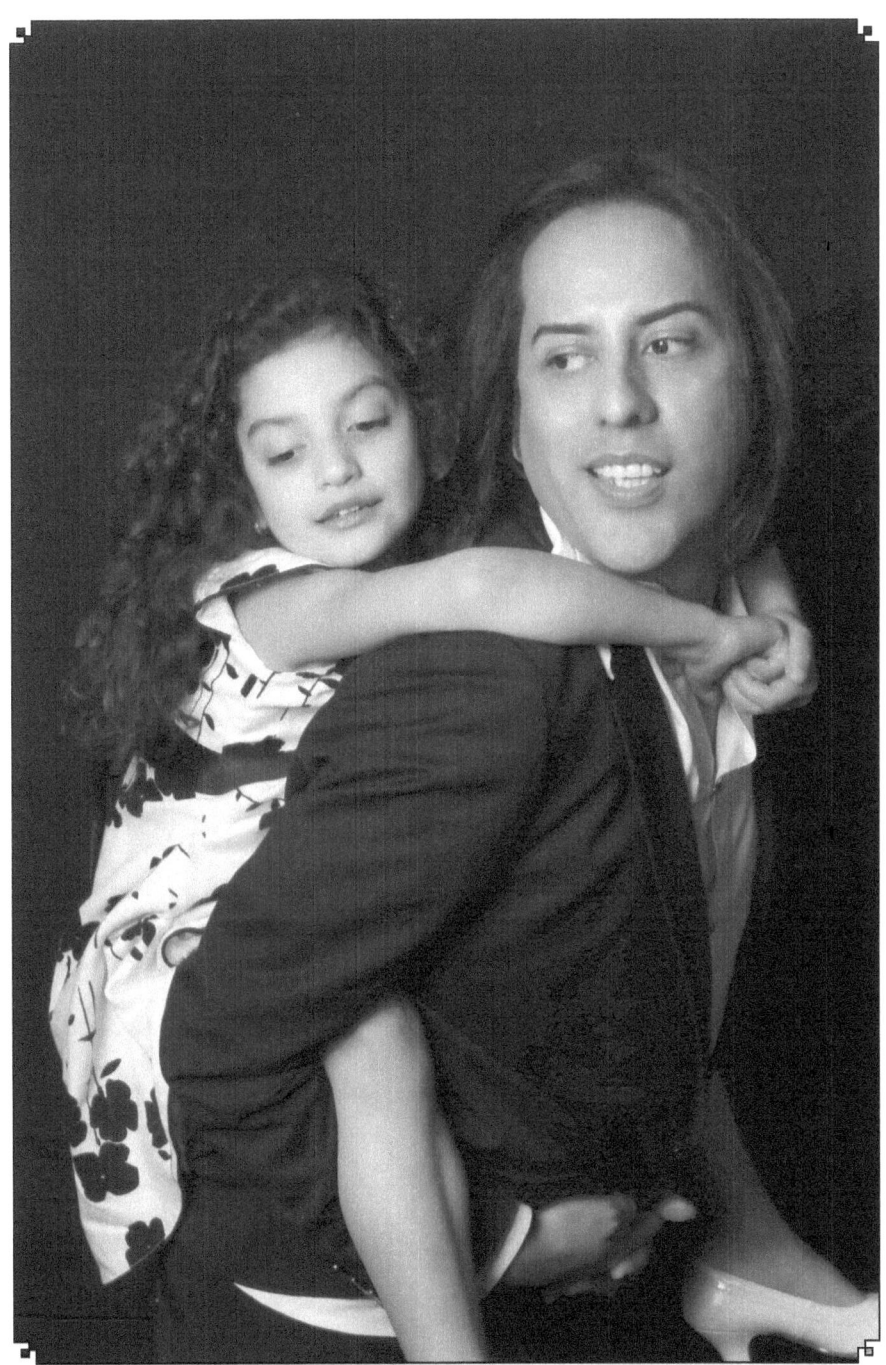

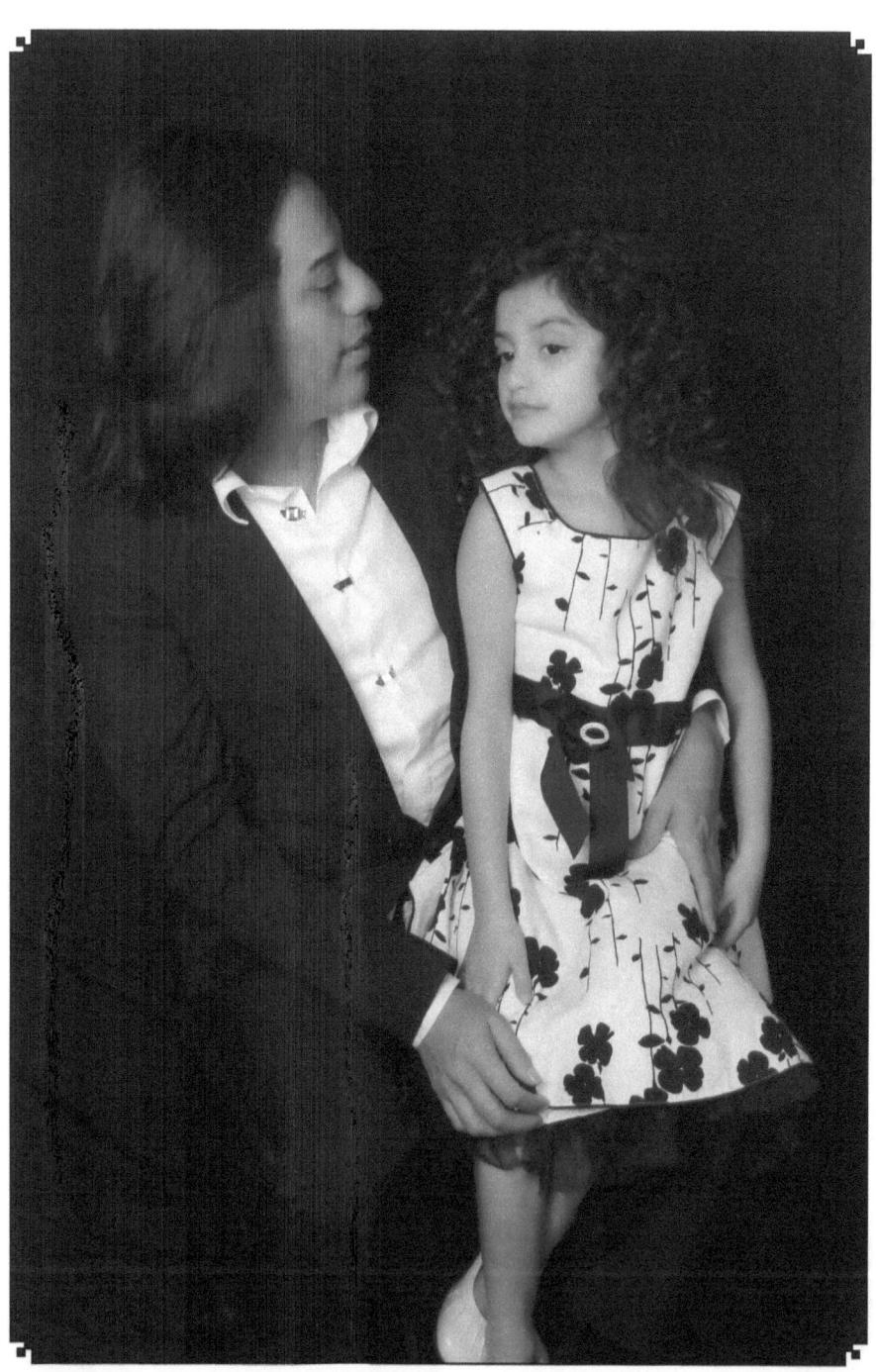

CHAPTER 16

Love

How many times have we tried to find the true meaning of love? Reading hundreds of pages that talk about it, establishing relationships and friendships, but none of them provide the exact meaning of this concept.

The definition of love is quite complicated, and we may safely say that there are two definitions, one technical and the other subjective, which can be created by you, according to your own values.

The correct or most accepted definition of the word love refers to a set of feelings that occur among people with the ability to develop emotions.

Love is a deep affection towards a person or a group of them, but not necessarily limited to address the human race, but includes those with whom we can develop emotional ties, such as your dog or any other pet, and indeed, even some material things.

Now it is vital that you learn to love yourself before you try to love anyone else, because otherwise you would not be giving true love to anyone, since you do not know what true love is.

To start it is necessary to accept who you are, with all your strengths and weaknesses, thanking the Universe for the wonder it has created in you. Self-respect and taking care of yourself in all aspects are the ultimate expressions of love.

An eight-year-old little girl who was returning home after school saw a sign at a House that said "Kittens for Sale". For the child, one of her life dreams was to own a kitten, so she went to the house to ask how much were the kittens.

Quickly she knocked on the door. A woman opened and asked: "How can I help you?" To which the girl replied: "How much are the kittens?"

The woman answered: "they are newborns and they cost ten dollars".

The child proposed a deal, and began to explain that her mother gave her a dollar every Sunday so that she could buy sweets, toys or any other thing that she wanted and that her biggest wish is to have a kitten, so she said: "Could I pay you a dollar every week until the ten dollars are paid? And until then could you give me the kitten?"

The woman could see the excitement in the little girl's small eyes and knew that she would be an excellent master that would take good care of the kitten without a doubt. It was then when the woman answered: "Let me propose another deal: I will give a kitten today in exchange that you come every Sunday and not miss paying me the dollar until you finish our deal." Then the woman asked the little girl to follow her to where she kept the kittens.

The child was filled with joy and excitement to see the number of beautiful kittens, but at the same time she noticed how one of the kittens was walking towards them with some difficulty and that it had a problem with one of its little legs. Immediately she picked him up and took him in her arms, saying: "I want this kitten, he's really cute." The woman was surprised and said, "that kitten is not worth anything, it was born with a defect in his leg and it can't run and play with you and much less make you happy."

The child, agitated, responded: "you don't know what you're talking about, this kitten is worth much more than any of the others and I'm going to show you why". The little girl crouched down and raised her long skirt up and showed the woman that she had a prosthetic leg saying, "I can't run or jump like other children either but I have a heart so big and full of love for humanity and for animals that is equal to or more than any other child in the world."

The woman felt ashamed and at the same time touched by the story of this child. She offered her apology and said, "Today I have learned a huge lesson that an eight year old has taught me." "The true value of people lies not in their limitations or in their physical appearance. It lies in their values as a human being".

Countless people choose, on their days off to not groom or to put on a nice ensemble, telling themselves that they will spend a relaxing and leisurely day, as no one important will come to visit.

What a wrong way of thinking. This is a living example of what it means to not give you the love that you deserve, just look at your reflection in the mirror and remember that you are the most important person in the universe.

There is a very unique and tender story that illustrates these concepts.

. . . .
LOVE
. . . .

Many years ago in a beautiful kingdom lived a newly married couple very much in love, a King and Queen. After some years the happy couple had the joy of becoming parents of two beautiful twin girls named Victoria and Elizabeth.

They were very dedicated to them from the beginning, giving them all their love in its various forms, from care, education, motivation and wellbeing that would definitely be reflected in both their health and their physical appearance at that time and in the future.

The beautiful princesses began to grow and were very beautiful and identical as two drops of clear and pure water. They participated in all activities, parties and were surrounded by the same people. As time passed each started to develop their own personality as is typical of people. Elizabeth was a beautiful girl on the outside but as far as her personality was concerned she found it hard to be sociable, didn't care much about her personal image as well as not being interested in stimulating herself intellectually. She had very little care not only with parents but with friends, even with her own sister. That caused people to slowly distance themselves from her without her realizing what was happening. Victoria was a girl always concerned about helping her community doing everything possible to help as needed. She had a very sweet demeanor and enjoyed reading, music and art. She loved her parents, friends, community and sister without taking into account the nature and form of the strange conduct of Elizabeth. Regarding her personality, she was very devoted to taking great care of her image always highlighting her natural beauty. She loved to take baths in the tub creating an ambiance with rich perfumes and adorning the room, with flowers and candles of subtle colors accompanied by soft calming music, seizing the moment to relax and reflect on her present and her future plans.

When they reached the age of eighteen the King and Queen organized a spectacular celebration. The party was attended by many young people of the girl's age. It was a night filled with music, delicious treats and surprises! It was a little strange to note how all the young men preferred dancing and conversing with Victoria. A very handsome young man was the center of attention that night because of his physical appearance and confident demeanor. That night the handsome young man took the decision to ask the lovely Elizabeth to dance when he noticed her all alone and distracted. They danced only one piece and the young man delicately walked her back to her seat, but she was extremely excited to have danced with the young man but he never noticed it because she did not reflect that emotion. Later, the handsome young man made the decision to ask Victoria to dance. They danced and danced through the night greatly enjoying it so much that the hours became seconds, they looked great together and the incredible chemistry between the two was obvious. From that night on they sealed a covenant of love which leads to the young man later asking Victoria's hand in marriage! Upon learning of this situation Elizabeth could not bear what was happening and asked the entire family why the young man had preferred her sister over her. The father overwhelmed and full of mixed feelings ordered a meeting in which the Queen, young daughters and a few of the young men who attended the party would participate. The next day all those called by the king to participate in the meeting came to the Kingdom.

The first thing the King did was to thank everyone for coming to the meeting then asked two of the young men what they thought about his daughters. The first said that both were equally beautiful but there was something that set them apart but he did not know how to describe it. The second agreed with what the first man said, but also added that despite both being equally beautiful physically, Elizabeth lacked a special glow that Victoria emitted but could not describe what that was exactly. Finally the King made a condition to the young man who had caused the controversy, he would need to give a good reason why he preferred Victoria and if it was good enough he would grant the marriage. The young man unhesitatingly started by saying that from a very young age he always admired both princesses and was well aware of their beauty, as well as their personalities. He then said he had always admired Victoria for since childhood she was known for being very friendly and attentive to all her family and her community helping and participating in charitable causes. Moreover it is a delight to talk with her because she had always been concerned about intellectual and spiritual preparation without forgetting her physical care. For me it is an example of what really is love. Love is seen, smelled, heard, savored but most importantly felt! She had shown the practice of all these actions. She has given us a living example to practice all these feelings that together are called Love. She loves herself and without fear of making a mistake she'll love me, and we will form a happy family!

When the young man finished his speech everyone stood up and applauded. Elizabeth clapped and then thanked him for the huge lesson about love to understand the importance of practicing all these feelings and promised to make the necessary changes to soon become a woman full of love and be happy!

Months after the majestic wedding was held they went on to live by practicing these beautiful set of feelings!

Never forget that true love is seen, smelled, heard, savored, but most importantly felt.

Love yourself!

Love is something you feel and you have to be sensitive to experience it!

CHAPTER 17

Love and parents

Love towards our parents is unconditional and infinite. We are products of love, and although in the course of our lives we reach certain differences, it is our responsibility to resolve those differences and reach a concrete agreement to make the relationship work between our parents and ourselves.

Remember that they gave you the greatest gift in the world, your being, and it is reflected in selfless love for you.

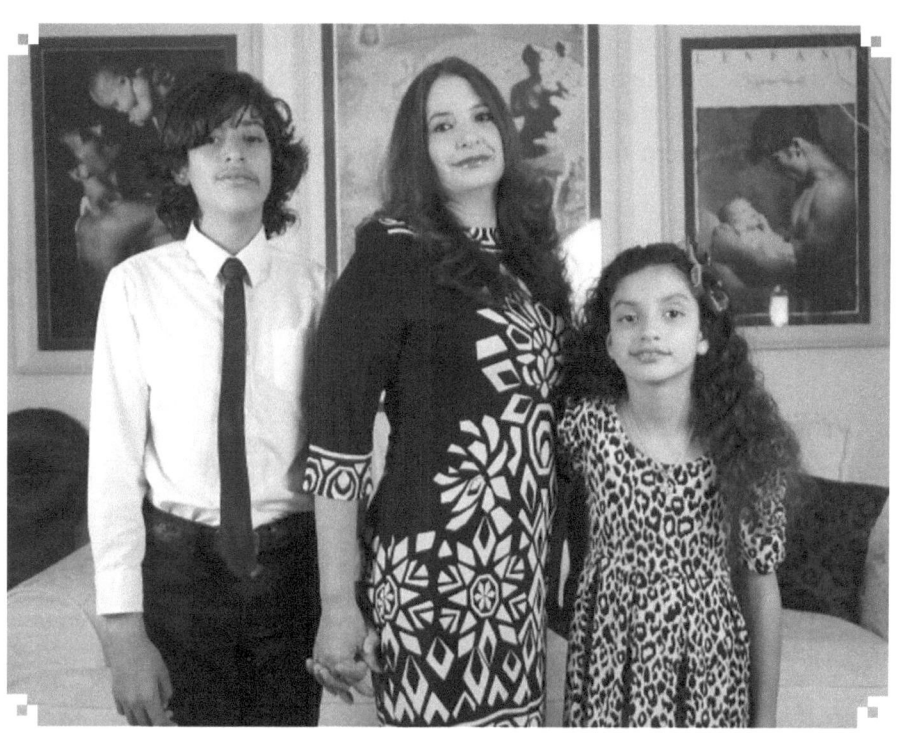

CHAPTER 18

Love towards our Mother

Without a doubt, love for our mother is the reflection of one of the greatest feelings, which is related to the fact that they carried us in their womb for nine months, not counting all the tenderness and care that they give us without expecting to receive any compensation for it.

Not only from our birth and childhood but also throughout our lives, because for her, no matter how old we are, we will always be her children.

The story I will tell you is about the lack of knowledge and sensitivity of one towards our mother.

LOVE TOWARD OUR MOTHER

Somewhere in the world a mother had two children; a fifteen year old and a six year old daughter. She carried out her tasks for the day, then looking at the clock she noticed that it was getting late to drop off her little one off at school. For this reason she decided to ask her eldest daughter to do her the favor of taking her sister, so that she could get there on time, but beforehand she sensed that at the time that she asked the favor, her daughter would give her a negative response.

Something typical for young people when they are in adolescence, they think that they have no responsibility at home and that only the mother had the obligation to do everything with the home.

The woman was hugely astonished to hear the positive answer from her daughter when asked and was surprised by it for a good while.

Later, the mother noticed that she didn't have enough bread for lunch and her husband was coming home to join them for lunch. It was then that she decided to venture and asked her daughter for another favor to go to the store to buy some bread.

She had a little bit of doubt of the response that her daughter would give her, so once again, she was surprised to hear a positive response from her daughter and that she also did it with great pleasure and without any problem or attitude.

While her daughter left the house, she raised her eyes towards heaven and started giving thanks because she thought that a divine power had touched this young lady making her an exemplary child and asked to never change her and to continue having this cooperative attitude at home.

In the evening, after finishing her duties, the mother was very tired; suddenly she recalled forgetting to wash the dishes after dinner, then decided to ask her daughter once again for her support to wash the dishes. She was sure of the answer, because she thought that from that day on things with her daughter would be great with this new spirit of cooperation, without suspecting that all this help had been conditional, since then her daughter had planned a strategy to solve her financial needs and get to go out with her friends, her boyfriend and other expenses that may come up later.

The daughter felt that her mother was always taking advantage of her by asking her for favors without giving her anything in return and this bothered her a lot. It was then that she decided to make an agreement with her, assuming that she would do it happily and would be in agreement and it would benefit them both.

So she wrote a letter that read:

Dear mother,

I know how hard you work at home and that you always need help. Today I propose to support you in whatever you need, as I did today, only to ask you for one thing in return, that you pay me to cover my personal expenses and whatever else that may come up. We will do it the following way:

For taking my sister to school this morning that's five dollars, for going to the store to buy bread that's another five dollars, washing the dishes from dinner, it's another five dollars; in total that's fifteen dollars. "Do you see? You help me and I help you and our problems are resolved."

She took the letter and placed it on the nightstand in her mother's bedroom before going to bed. She left her door slightly open to see the reaction that her mother would have after reading her letter.

A few moments later she saw her mother come out of her room with a very sad look and tears running down her face. Immediately the daughter assumed that their parents had an argument as they would do normally, and that she had not even taken notice of her letter, much less had she thought about reading it, so she came to the conclusion that her plan had failed and that things would remain the same.

She closed the door being annoyed and decided to sleep. When she woke up the next morning, she noticed that there was an envelope and opened it happily thinking that her mother had accepted her proposal.

Upon opening it, she found fifteen dollars, as well as a note that read:

Dear daughter:

I thank you with all my heart all that you did for me yesterday. I only want to say something to you that is very important that you should know: by having you in my belly with much love for nine months, for taking care of you, in your time of need when sick, feeding you, giving you a home, for providing your education and for worrying about you every moment and of every day of your life and above all, for giving you life and loving you until my dying day, you don't owe me anything.

Sincerely,

"Your mother who loves you unconditionally"

The young lady felt like her heart dropped, her body contorting and her eyes watering as they shed endless tears.

Without hesitating, she ran to embrace her mother, apologizing for her poor attitude and thanking her for everything she did, especially for the greatest lesson of love that she will never forget.

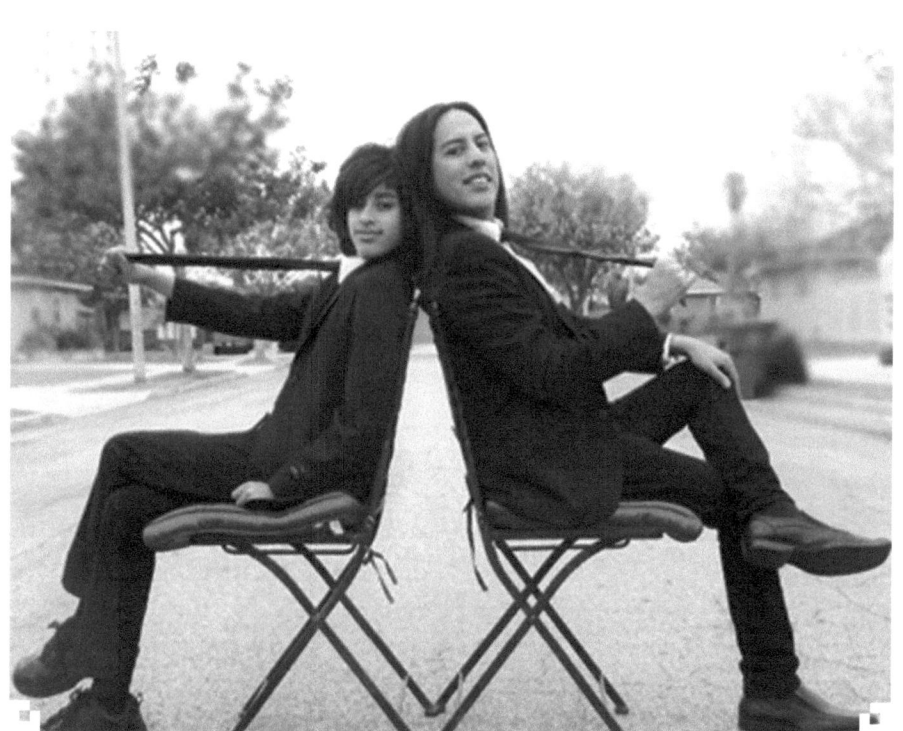

CHAPTER 19

Love towards our Father

This type of love is not less than that of the mother. They are simply different ways of loving each one of them. The coexistence that we have with the people around us during our life depends on the closeness that we have with them.

The love of the father is also essential in the development and growth of each of us. It is our source of inspiration and a pattern to follow in life, from this depends much our forming as individuals. We imitate his actions and reactions, his image is often visualized as that of a man of strict rules and strong feelings, but in him dwells a sensitive soul full of affection, love and tenderness. Those feelings stand out more when life gives him the wonderful opportunity to be a father.

As my grandfather used to tell me; "You are not a son until you are a parent".

A story tells, of a distant city of Mexico in the garden of a house where there was a beautiful peach tree. In that house lived a couple with a small five year old girl. The child enjoyed playing around the tree, often climbing it, until after a while her father made her a treehouse and it laid on top of the leafy branches.

The girl played in the treehouse every day or whenever she had the opportunity. The girl loved the tree intensely, not only because she played in the treehouse or because she would eat from its delicious peaches, but because of the loving bond that existed between her and the tree.

Over the years the girl became a woman and moved to a different city. Later, she went back to visit the tree who was happy to see her and said: "How wonderful to see you again, have you come to play with me", to which the woman replied: "No, I'm very sad because I need money for my children, and I have none." The tree happily replied, "Do not worry, cut and sell all my peaches, so you may purchase toys and have money for whatever else you need for your children." The woman left happy.

The years passed and the tree thought of the woman and how she had not come to visit.

Later, she came back again, and the tree, excited in her presence, asked: "Have you come to play with me?" To which the woman replied: "No, I'm very sad because I need a house for my family, can you help me?" The tree unhesitatingly replied smiling, "Cut my branches and build the house for your family", so the woman cut off the branches and left happily.

Ten years passed and the tree was saddened by the thought of the child who gave him so much happiness and whom he missed.

Again, the woman came back to visit the tree and the tree repeated again the same question "Are you coming to play with me?" To which the woman replied: "I can't play with you, I'm sad and I'm getting old. I want a rocking chair, can you give me one?" The tree said, "Use my trunk to build one so you can rest and be happy." The woman cut the trunk and went away for a long time.

Finally, after many years she returned and the tree said, "I'm sorry, but I have nothing else to give, not even peaches."

The woman replied, "I have no teeth to bite, nor strength to climb, I do not need much now, I just want a place to rest, because I'm old and tired after so many years."

The tree, touched by what the woman said, replied: "I have nothing more to give you, the only thing left are my dying roots, but old tree roots are the best place to lie down and rest. Sit down with me and rest." The woman sat by the tree, and the tree happy and content, smiled with tears in his eyes.

This story could be that of any of us. The tree is our parents, and as children we love them and play with them.

When we grow up we forget about them and only return when we need something or we're in trouble, and no matter what it is, they will always be there to give us all they can just to see us happy.

It seems that the girl in this story is cruel to the tree, as we are when we mistreat our parents. Value and revere your parents. Make them happy and enjoy them while you have them with you.

CHAPTER 20

Love towards our children

This love starts from the beginning of pregnancy, and grows daily, waiting for the baby's arrival. It continues and intensifies over seeing them born, grow and develop. Such is the passion and devotion for them, that we are capable of doing the impossible, to the point of giving our life for them.

Let's remember that a father is not the one who births, but the one who raises and shapes the child so I mean this feeling is also given, in the same way, in cases of people who adopt a child, no matter if the child is not the product of a marriage.

It is said that a couple arrived at the hospital desperate and agitated. When meeting face to face with the doctor who treated their daughter they asked him "How is our daughter Patricia? They said she worsened ", to which the doctor replied," I'm sorry, we did everything that we could, we lost the battle to leukemia"

The parents cried desperately. The doctor allowed them to enter the room to be with their daughter for a moment. The girl's wish was to donate her organs to the hospital to save the lives of other children.

After some time, the nurse on duty came into the room and said: "Sir, Mam, its time". The parents wept inconsolably, it was then the nurse asked if they wanted a lock of her hair to keep together with all hers belongings, to which they responded affirmatively. The nurse cut the hair lock and placed it inside a plastic bag along with all her other belongings.

The parents went on their way home crying. Arriving at their residence, it was so difficult for them to enter the room of the child, they both sat down on her bed, breathing in the scent of the child.

They cried themselves to sleep. Later, upon waking, they noticed that on the pillow there was an envelope. The mother quickly opened it and read the letter which was written by the girl:

"Dear parents,

Do not be sad, I am very well, I have come to this wonderful paradise now and I no longer have Leukemia. I have my hair and my nails again. My grandparents welcomed me and they have led me to explore this beautiful place.

That Wonderful Being that everyone speaks of took me by the hand and sat me on his lap. I recognized him by the images depicted of him on Earth.

He told me to be calm and worry free, he invited me to dinner tonight, he gives me an incredible spiritual peace and I asked if I was allowed to write a letter. Then he himself lent me his pen and gave me paper.

Dad, Mom, I propose that you adopt a child she will make you very happy. Also she can use my room and my toys. A boy may not be a good idea he will not like my toys. Rest assured, I am very happy.

Well now I have to go, I just want you to remember that although I'm not physically present, my spirit will always be with you and I will always love you.

I say goodbye because I have to return the pen that He let me borrow, he has to keep writing in his book the names of more children who are on their way to be born.

I will love you forever,

Patricia

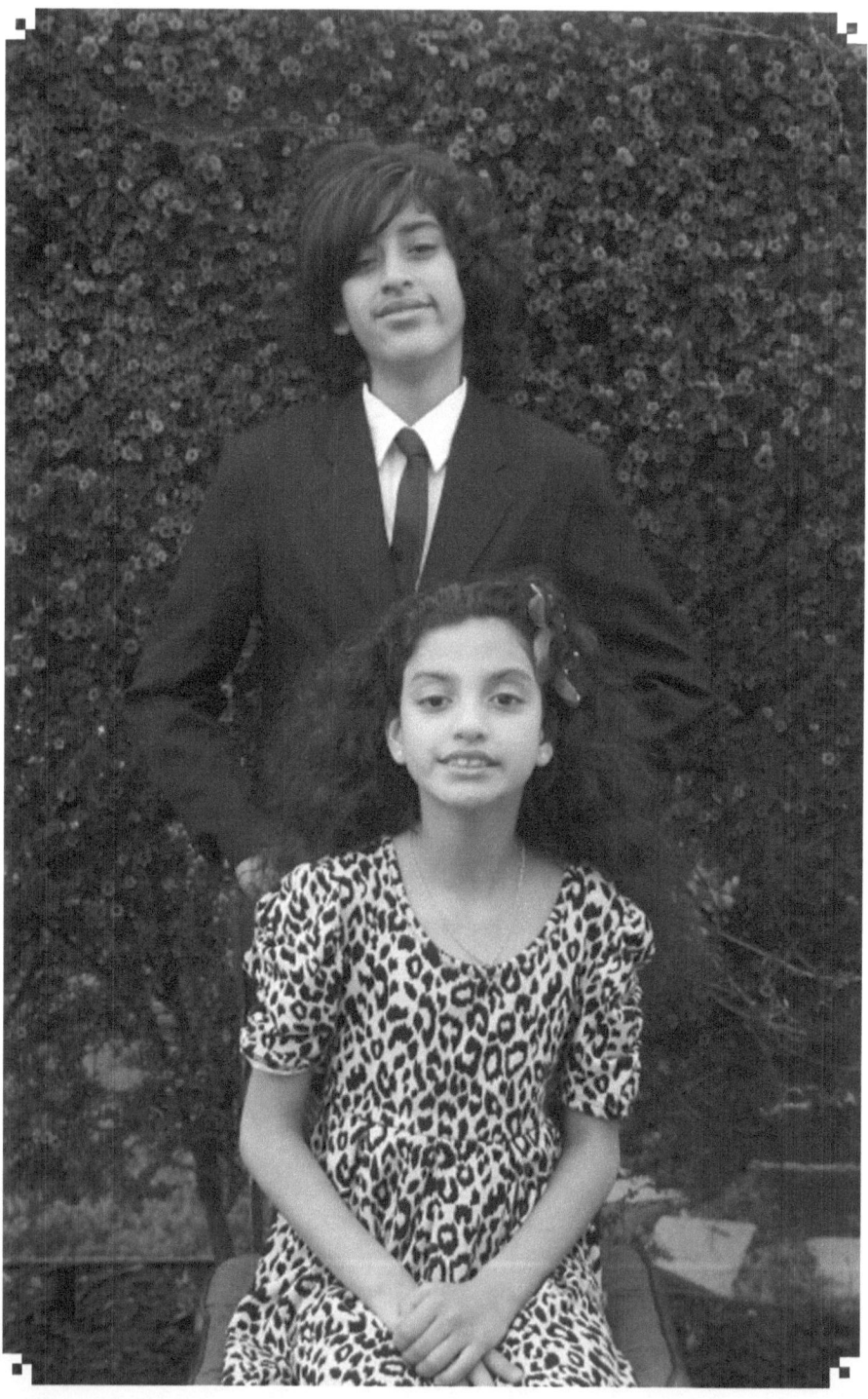

CHAPTER 21

Love towards Siblings

This kind of love is very particular, simply for the reason that they carry the same blood.

Born by the seed of love that sprouts between a couple, which eventually grows and enlarges by coexisting with each other.

Surely during growth there will be brawls, arguments, disagreements and problems that will be solved due to the love that unites them. I have heard of many stories where siblings have come to have very serious problems, to the point of wishing each other death. I never could understand how it is that people who carry the same blood can reach that point, perhaps a result of poor communication, lack of humility and above all the absence of values.

If you ever get to live situations that separate you from your siblings, I suggest you take some time to think things better so you can see more clearly the problem, then, seek your sibling and resolve the situation as soon as you can. Believe me, if you let time pass, it may be too late and maybe when you finally decide to resolve the issue, life may not give you that opportunity and your sibling may no longer be within your reach.

Two brothers were walking on the beach sand, having a conversation about a certain topic. There was a moment during the conversation where they disagreed and everything turned into an argument.

The one who was not right indeed got very angry. Such was his anger that he gave his brother a hard slap.

Feeling beat, the other brother just reacted calmly and quietly continued his walk.

They later decided to swim in the ocean. The brother who had launched the slap had trouble swimming and as a consequence he began to drown. His brother without thinking, went to his aid and acted skillfully and quickly to keep him from drowning until he was safe on the sand. Once he recovered they continued their walk, when suddenly the brother said, "I want to apologize for having assaulted you even though I was not right in that discussion, and at the same time I feel very confused because there are two things I do not understand." "Why after I gave you a slap unfairly, you saved my life?" "I also wonder why after the pain I caused you, you wrote on the sand but the action you took to save my life you carved onto a rock!" To which the brother replied, the bad things that happen in my life I always write them on the sand, for when the wave of oblivion washes upon the sand it deletes them. But the beautiful things in life that happen to me, I always record them on the rocks as a lasting beautiful memory for all my life.

An Old Legend

An old legend has it that a beautiful couple months after marriage were blessed to get pregnant. Emotions grew immediately. The man looked after and spoiled his beloved knowing how important being in a good mood was. They anxiously awaited the arrival time of their baby. She ate very healthy and cared for their home just as well. After she completed chores at home she took time to knit clothes for her future baby in neutral colors since she had no idea if their child would be a boy or a girl. The only thing she wanted was for the children to be born strong and healthy. The couple lived day to day happily to see how her stomach grew imagining what life has in store for them. After all the waiting the woman began to feel pain immediately knowing they were typical signs of going into labor. This happened during the night and while her husband slept. The labor pains sharpened and the woman awoke her husband and they rushed to the hospital without any clues about the new life that would come in a few hours. After a while in the hospital, she finally gave birth. That was when life gave them a great surprise to find that they had given birth to two beautiful boys Mark and Sebastian. The children were very healthy and as time passed and the family of four lived in harmony and happiness. When Mark and Sebastian turned eight their parents discovered that again they were expecting another baby and as a birthday gift made the announcement to their children without suspecting that it would cause jealousy for both children. Thereafter the issue became very uncomfortable to the children and the parents. When it finally came time for the birth of the baby they left the Grandma in charge of the children. Happy and nervous the couple went to the hospital to give birth and, that was when life gave them one more surprise. The new baby was a beautiful girl which they named Cecille. The parents were convinced that Cecille would not cause any jealousy for their children being that she was the little girl. They would see things differently and not as competition but the opposite would happen and they would care, protect and love which did not happen. They grew a strange jealousy. They always tried to stay out of what was happening with Cecille, avoiding the thing that caused pain and sadness to the child and parents. While preparing a beautiful party for Cecille for her fifteenth birthday, the brothers planned to scare her. They never imagined that they would send her to the hospital on the brink of death. Cecille was in the hospital, bedridden with the parents close by feeling terribly sad and depressed. When Mark and Sebastian arrived ashamed and sad at what they had caused. A few seconds later the doctor on duty arrived and said; "Gentlemen you must be strong and keep the faith because only a miracle can save this young woman". The family hugged while the doctor departed. A few minutes later Mark asked to join hands to form a circle around Cecille. Remembering mother saying that in tough times she taught them the power of prayer and faith and asked them to join together their faith and prayers to achieve recovery of their sister. Sebastian took the floor and said; "before starting I would like to ask for Mark's and my forgiveness from Cecille, we are very sorry and ashamed for all of this misery we caused and we love you with all our hearts". He immediately held hands and began to pray they did so for several minutes at the end were silent but continued holding hands. To his surprise Cecille opened her eyes and smiled with a few tears in her eyes began telling her family I love you all and would not trade you for anybody else. She rose up and they all hugged. The doctor gave a cheer and said; "what has happened is a true miracle". The father added; "yes Dr. a miracle from the blood and love between siblings!"

From that day forward Cecille simply became Princess Cecille. They lived the rest of their lives happily learning and remembering that blood is unique and that love for the brethren is forever!

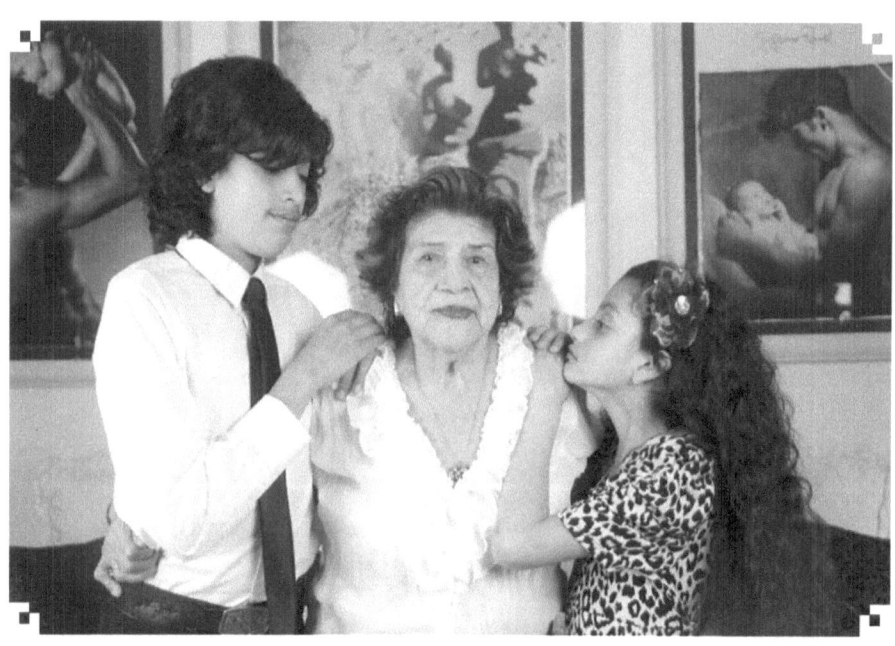

CHAPTER 22

Love towards our grandparents

How to bypass a love so tender and so special, if it is basically where a great love story begins, which results in the existence and future love between our parents.

They truly deserve a tribute for they are carriers of great stories and traditions that transcend our days.

It is said that their love towards us is very similar to the love of our parents and even their passion can get to be so much, that they become our accomplices in some of our shenanigans as children, in our confidents as adolescents and our support as adults.

Allow me to tell you about a story of a friend of mine. His name is Kenny Bernazar.

On a Saturday night when we were getting ready to leave for an event, I could see a change in his behavior. His eyes looked sad and he seemed very thoughtful, which is why I asked: "What's the matter, are you having problems my friend? May I help you with anything? To which he replied; "My friend, I feel very sad, remember I told you that, not having my father beside me since I was born, my grandfather was the one who took the responsibility for my family and helped my mother with everything she needed?"

"The image I remember of my grandfather is the image of a tall, strong man, full of energy and lots of love to give." Every day he gave himself the task of taking me to school and picking me up. We played together 'till we would die of laughter. He always had time for me. During very special moments he told me his stories and it would take me back to his days of youth. It was fascinating."

"How could I forget that? Well, the years have passed and this morning I went to visit him. To go into his room and watch him in bed felt very sad. There was not even a shadow of what he once was ". The years and his diseases have deteriorated him. He does not smile like before, nor does he tell me his stories. I feel that the time is close and soon he will no longer be with me." Tears rolled down his cheeks, so I said, "My friend, do not be sad. Re-live all those great memories of your childhood. Change sadness for a deserved tribute to him. This is when it is your turn to take care of him, give him all your love, affection, patience and understanding to provide him happiness, precisely now that he is alive, so that when he has to leave to his final destination, you're calm and at peace for having returned a little of all the love he gave you during his existence."

Keep in mind that we were all children at one point then young men and we will at one point be old.

A man who had dedicated his life to work hard to give his family everything they needed, had only one son, living in a very beautiful large house full of luxuries, and his wife. He and his wife were the perfect couple. Over the years their small child had become a man, the pride of his father, an exemplary university student.

One day he decided to marry his beautiful girlfriend, and years later they conceived a child who his grandfather adored, he was all joy and made him feel like he was living a second youth.

Time passed and the little boy's grandmother died, his grandfather being alone in his big house was sad, too sad. One afternoon while sitting on his favorite chair an idea came to the grandfather's mind, he then decided to go visit his son, when he knocked on the door it was his ten year old grandson who attended the door and immediately hugged him, giving him a strong kiss, and full of happiness invited him in.

In the living room was his son, who greeted him and soon they started a conversation. The grandfather took advantage of the chat to tell his son about an idea he had, and said, "You know son, since the death of your mother I feel very lonely and sad. This afternoon while taking a break and relaxing, an idea came to my mind I would like to share with you."

"You live in a big house with many rooms, and I thought I'd ask if I could come live with you the last few years I have left of life, to enjoy you, my daughter-in-law and, most importantly, my grandson." The man immediately replied, "Father, it is true that I have many rooms in this house, but I have guests that stay in them very often, so it would bother me if you would come to live in this house."

The grandfather lowered his head, and as his eyes watered and he said, "You're very right my son."

They had not realized that the ten year old boy was listening to the conversation, the child without thinking twice told his father; "Dad, I have a solution; my room is large, we could add a bed that my grandfather could occupy." His father replied, "Son, you do not know what you're saying, maybe this idea may work for a while, but when you get older you will need your privacy, then your grandfather would become a nuisance."

The boy could not help being sad at such a response. Then the grandfather said; "my son, I just remembered something, you have a garage with space for four cars, yours, your wife's and the luxury car so there is space left. If you'll allow it, I could take that space, I certainly will not bother you, nor will I give you any problems."

The son had no choice but to accept and asked the child to go to the linens closet and bring a blanket for his grandfather who for that night on would live with them.

The child obeyed the order, but took a while. Meanwhile the grandfather was talking to his son. The man showed a bored face because he didn't find the conversation interesting with his father.

When the boy returned, his father struck him with the question of why he had taken so long and said, "Your grandfather must be tired and has to go to sleep"! The boy replied; "It took me long because I went for a pair of scissors." The father asked "scissors, what for?" "Yes, dad, I needed them to cut the blanket in two parts". The father asked, "Why did you cut the blanket?" The boy replied: "I cut it to use one part for my grandfather, and one I will keep for when your time comes, my father."

What a lesson for all.

Remember it only takes a blink of an eye for ten, twenty years to go by, for sooner or later we will all grow old.

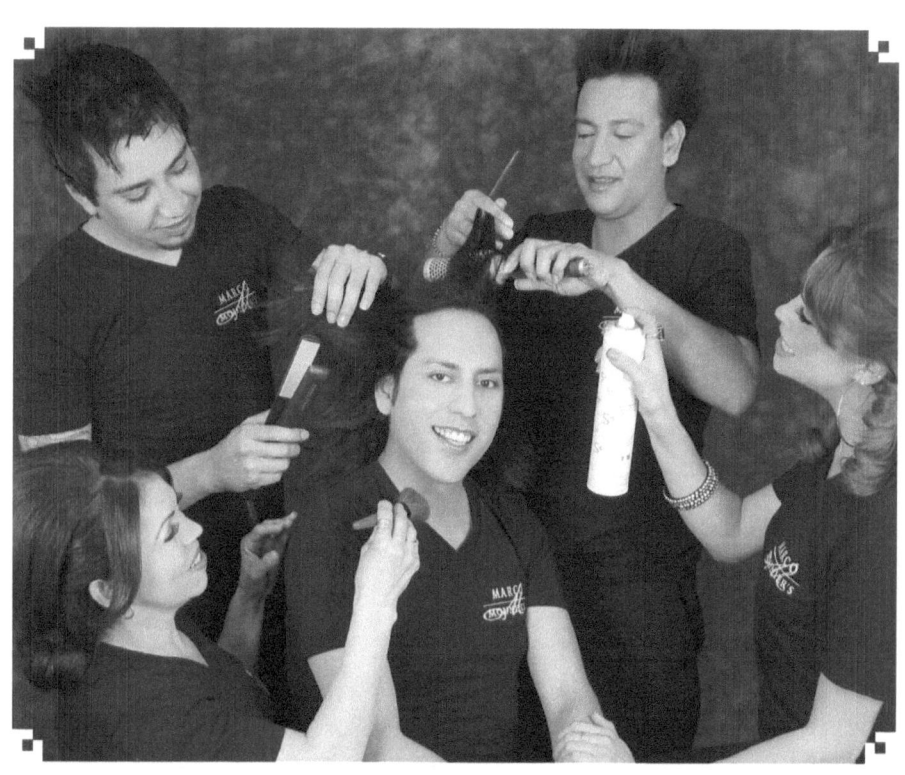

CHAPTER 23

Love towards Friends

We plant a seed, and how we care for it determines how beautiful that plant can become. It all starts when you meet a person with whom, by his behavior, attitudes and other details, we have a special approach, giving a feeling that we can identify with.

Friendship should be based on honesty and love for others. A true friend will not be precisely the one who always tells you you're right, but one who is sincere and honest with you, letting you know when you make a mistake, reprimanding you and calling to your attention when you're not doing something right.

Some friends even feel more as if they were your siblings. A true friend is not necessarily the one you talk to or visit daily, rather it is one that, despite having spent time apart, when they meet you again, it seems that time did not pass by, even though there was no contact. Cultivate a friendship.

A king and queen, who lived in a beautiful castle, saw the birth of their daughter, a beautiful princess, for whom her parents did everything to give her the best, for she was the pride of the couple.

Years passed, and one afternoon, while talking the king and queen noted that their daughter had reached the age of marriage. In agreement, they decided to announce that they would seek the perfect candidate for their daughter to contract nuptials.

The announcement was made in general regardless of whether the candidate belonged to royalty or not. The requirement was that whoever wanted to marry her would need to be an honest man, with moral values and above all the desire to make her very happy.

The king prepared a number of pots in which he planted a seed that each of the participants had to cultivate, giving it all the care and love needed in order to grow a beautiful plant. He ordered to each of the candidates to take a pot and take it home to begin their work. He had also set a time for them to return to show the results.

After this time, all participants went on their way back to the castle. There was only one young man who was very upset and was telling his mother that he would not go to the meeting saying; "Dear Mother, I feel very embarrassed. I gave the seed all the love and care necessary to see the seed germinate into a beautiful plant, but I got absolutely nothing." The mother said; "you've always been a perfect son, a great friend and above all a human being with great values. Do not worry, take the pot that the king gave you and present it to him."

The young man went to the castle. On the way he met several of the candidates who made fun of him, because they saw the result, unlike theirs, who had beautiful small trees and other plants with colorful flowers.

Finally, being all together in the castle, the king came down to see the results of each candidate for himself. He became increasingly more and more surprised when suddenly he found the young man whose seed had not germinated and watched his face with embarrassment and his eyes filled with sadness.

At that time the king stood up, and loudly announced, "Ladies and Gentlemen, I am proud to present to you the new prince of this kingdom, the man who will be the husband of my daughter." The surprised young man said; "my king, why your decision? I was not able to make this seed germinate despite all the affection and love that I offered it." The king, announced loudly; "in each of the pots I had planted a sterile seed, therefore, if you had all been honest, none of you would have brought any type of plant, but this young man was the only honest person, he had the courage to come here, to introduce his result, which is such an act of honesty and values, I am sure he will be able to love and make my princess very happy."

Honesty is certainly one of the greatest virtues that man must have and is part of every relationship, without exception.

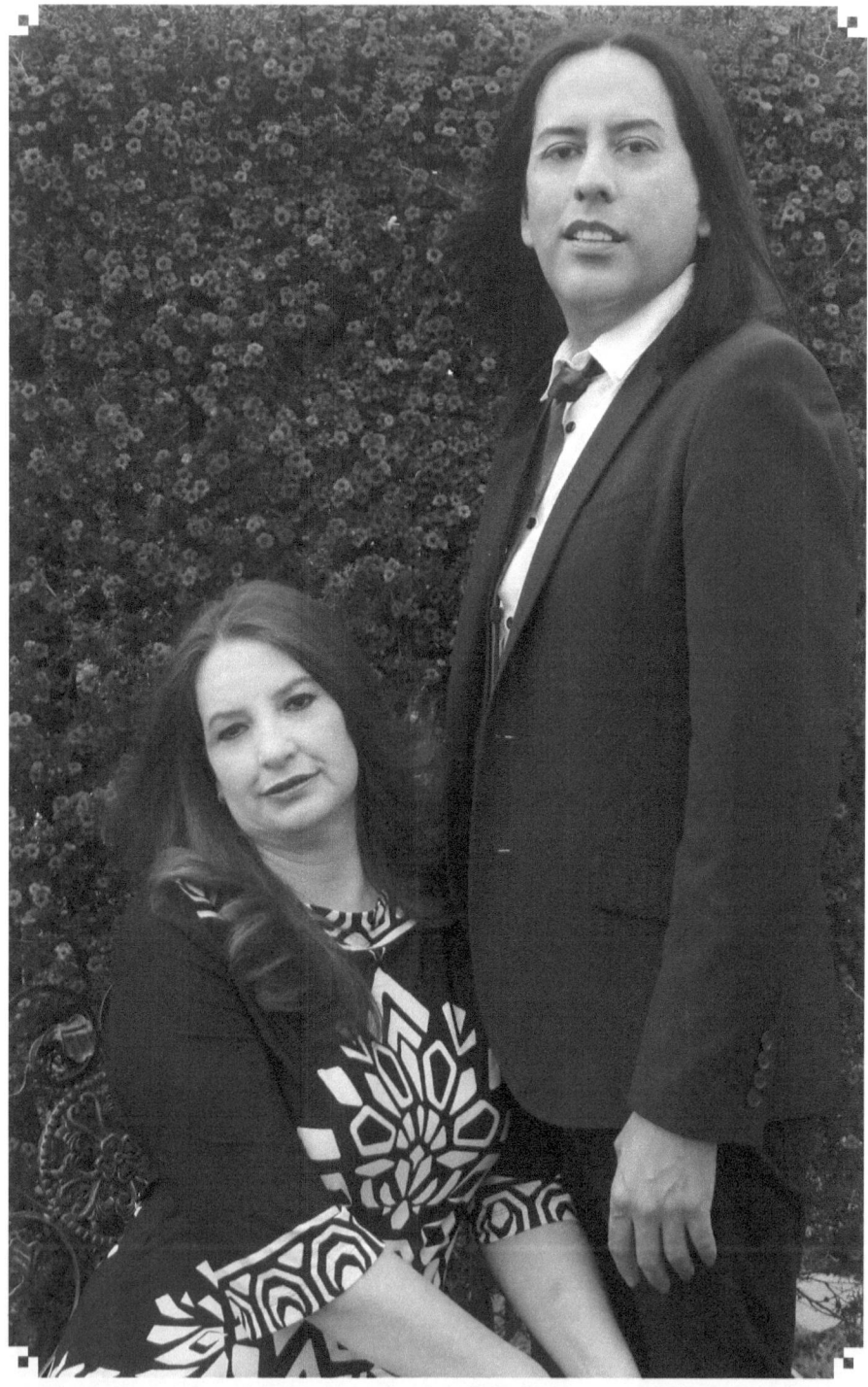

CHAPTER 24

Love towards our Partner

An entire range of feelings form a couple's true love, ranging from physical attraction, treatment and details, until achieving compatibility.

Although always so controversial and often complicated, basically because we provoke it, this kind of love begins with an unexpected tender look, or an unprepared meeting, although sometimes a relationship may be through dealing with the person, physical contact and the coexistence, and as in all types of couples, sharing an interest for various activities.

When I talk about the controversial, I refer to that stage in which there begins to be differences in couples and we notice the famous incompatibility.

How often I have heard people talk about their search, or as many say, they have found the one.

Later, after the success proclaimed to have found their better half, problems arise which sometimes cannot be overcome due to the lack of communication and above all by the desire to reach a settlement based on the great love that brought them together in the beginning.

Up to this point I could not understand the phrase "looking for my other half" or "I have found my other half", when the reality is there is no such thing. I proved it in my relationship, because if it was about the other half, my partner would be a watermelon and I would be a cantaloupe, because the truth is we don't fit each other as halves. She is so different than me, though many things are very similar, and it is this combination that has given us success in our relationship, along with communication, respect, prudence, admiration, patience, and above all, the commitment that unites us.

This time I want to tell two stories regarding couples, and to tell the truth it was quite difficult to choose among several of the most interesting and beautiful love stories.

. . . .

The Beggar and the Queen

. . . .

In a great castle lived a beautiful Queen, one day she realized that despite having everything that apparently made her happy, her heart felt empty, for lack of a mate and it was then that she decided to announce her desire to marry.

It had to be with a man who could prove that he would make her happy. Many handsome men attended, offering the Queen everything from gorgeous smiles and striking eyes, to sexy and strong physique.

After a while, they announced that a beggar asked to be considered and wished to talk to her. When the man finally arrived where the Queen sat, he said; "Dear Queen, I have nothing to offer, only a true love and an infinite admiration for your majesty that was born within me since childhood and I wholeheartedly wish to be your husband, so I want to make a proposal. "I will ascend to the highest tower of the castle, and sit on the balcony for ninety days. I will be exposed to inclement weather, rain, sun, dust, but even more… I shall suffer from thirst and hunger, if after those hundred days, I manage to resist then that will be my concrete proof of love towards you. Then I will become your husband and the King." The Queen strongly surprised by such a proposal, accepted.

The beggar rose to the highest tower and sat on the balcony. Time ran

and the man held his proposal, it had been eighty-nine days, eleven hours and thirty minutes, the people gathered outside the castle, and after all this time they were happy because they assumed that this man would be the new King.

They all counted the minutes so that eventually, they would have a grand celebration. The beggar looked broken, deteriorated, and weak with sad eyes.

Just as the time had passed and were now eighty-nine days, eleven hours and forty five minutes, you could hear the bustle and happiness of the whole kingdom.

Suddenly the man announced that he would give up. Not caring about anything he stood up and headed home. When he arrived, the first thing he faced was his mother, who once finding out of the situation and could not leave behind her astonishment and rebuked him: "I cannot understand what happened. How is it that after enduring all this time, and when the whole kingdom was taking for granted that you would be the new King, you decided to consider yourself defeated. Can you tell me why you gave up?"

"Dear mother," he began to explain, "I was for eighty nine days, eleven hours and forty-five minutes on her balcony, supporting all such calamities, and meanwhile, she could not show even a bit of pity for my suffering. I waited all this time for a sign of goodness and consideration that never came. So I realized that a person so selfish, inconsiderate and blind, who just thinks about themselves does not deserve my love."

When you love someone and you feel that for that person to be by your side you need to suffer, sacrifice your essence and get to the point of begging, even if it hurts, walk away. Not just because things become difficult, but because that someone who doesn't make you feel valued, will never be capable of giving you the same in return. Those who do not give in with the same commitment do not deserve you.

• •

The Hawk and the Seagull

• •

A couple, who swore they had found love at first sight, would call themselves the perfect match. They wanted to spend the rest of their lives together, free of problems, disagreements and sad moments that may cause separation and decided to go to a sorcerer, who was known as the best in the world.

Upon arriving to the home of the sorcerer, they asked him for a spell to ensure that they would always be together until the day of their death, for they infinitely loved each other.

To perform the spell, the sorcerer asked the woman to go in search of the most beautiful seagull she could find, one that would fly as high as possible, exuding freedom. As for the man he asked to find and bring a beautiful hawk which would be strong and would fly the highest possible exuding freedom.

Aware of what the wizard had asked, they left, turning to the task of finding what was needed to make the spell that would allow them to stay together for the rest of their lives.

Weeks later they managed to find and bring the birds back to the sorcerer. The excited woman and man asked, "What will you do with them? Will you kill them to make this spell? Will you bathe us in their blood so we may always be together?" The Sorcerer, without answering these questions, asked them to tie the hawk and the seagull by the legs, using a rope he provided.

The shocked couple followed the directions of the wizard, who then said; "Now that you have them securely fastened by the legs, throw them up in the air and let them fly as high as they can and live their lives."

As soon as they launched them up in the air, they watched how they fell to the ground and immediately began to attack each other for they felt tied and unable to fly as high as they were accustomed to.

The couple, terrified at such an event, asked the wizard, "What is happening?" The sorcerer replied; "This is the result of the spell that you have asked me to do for you."

The couple asked: "Can you tell us clearly what your words mean?" He said; "The birds, feeling tied, fought for their freedom, as happens when a couple truly loves each other, you do not need to have your future secured through a spell to be together, you both must learn to keep your individuality, giving each other all the support love you need and maintaining communication between the two of you. Fly as high as you wish individually to achieve your personal goals and ideals, so you may be happy and make your partner happy."

The couple left thanking the sorcerer for such a magnificent lesson. Ensuring him they had learned that all human beings as individuals must fly as high as they want, drawing their own paths, fighting to achieve happiness, and at the same time, progress together, respecting their space and helping each other achieve personal success individually and then success as a couple.

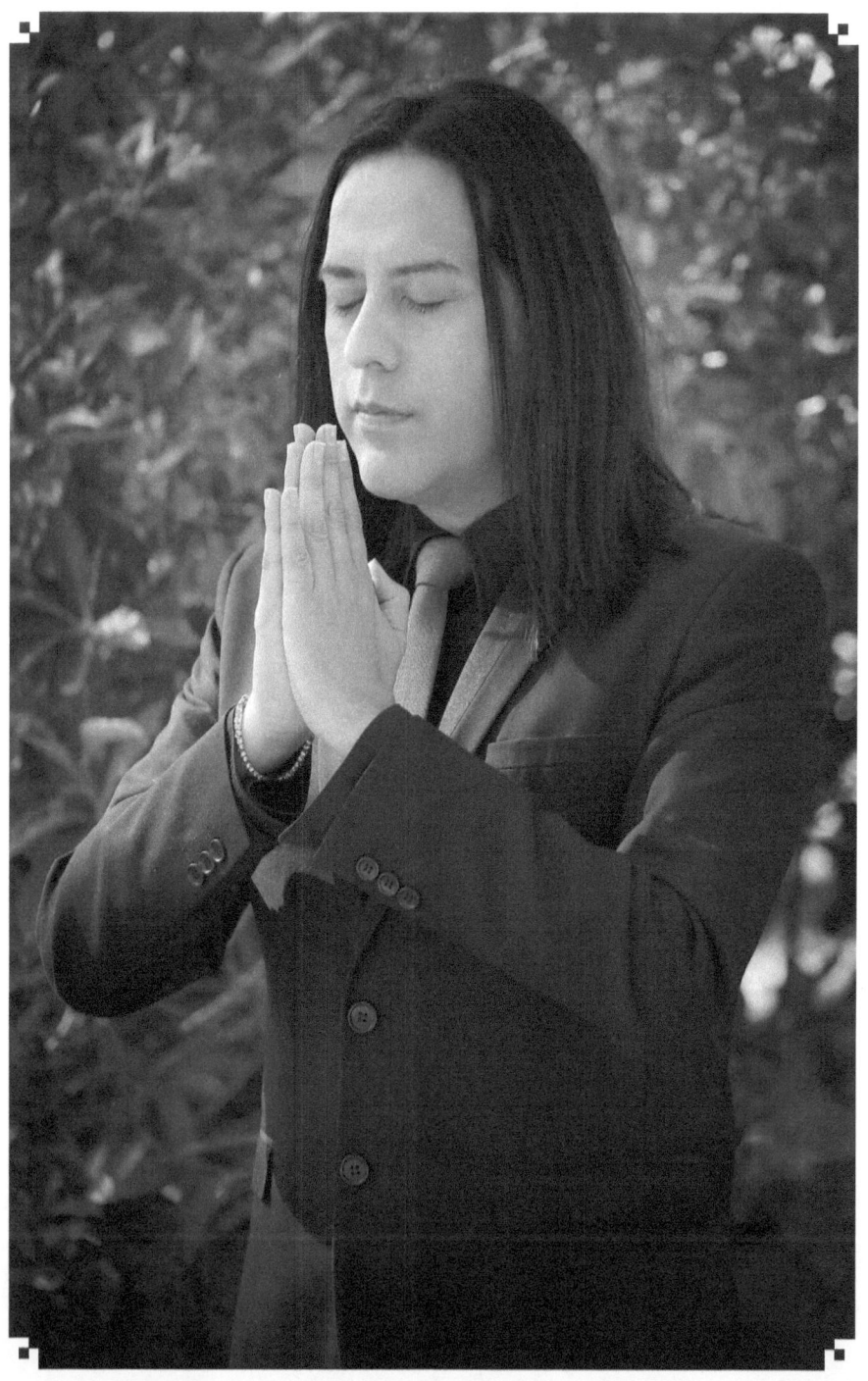

CHAPTER 25

Forgiveness

Forgiveness is a great manifestation of love. The lack of it poisons the soul drop by drop, takes away your peace and interrupts your minds tranquility, robs you of sleep and visibly affects your physical appearance.

Forgiveness does not mean to stop caring about what happened, or much less to agree with someone who hurt you.

Forgiveness is letting go of all that hurts you, to feel released. By forgiving you do not do a favor to someone else but for yourself.

Many times, the most important person you have to forgive is yourself, for all the things you did or did not do. Forgiveness is an acknowledgment that you have the duty of renewing every day.

I wish you all the happiness in the world.

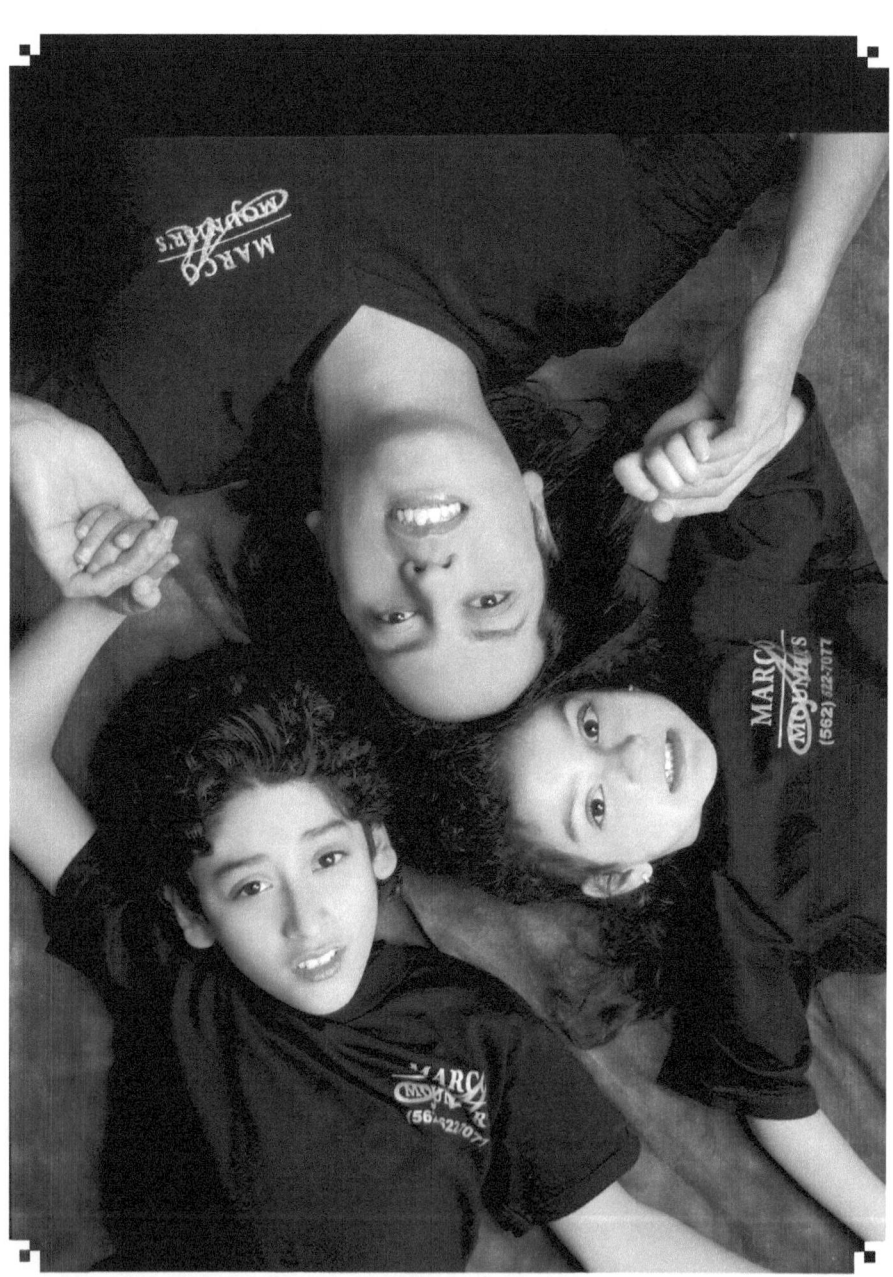

CHAPTER 26

Love and the Universe

Love is born. Without a doubt, it is the most beautiful feeling of all, the mirror of the soul that makes us touch happiness and we must practice it every day and share it with our loved ones, starting with the ones at home.

We must create light in the home and outside of the home. May our words be a reflection of our deeds, may it arise from the depths of us like the scent that a flower distills, like the kiss of a baby, like the shelter of a mother who consoles and comforts us even during the most difficult moments of life.

Love is a passage to paradise and we as humans must understand that we carry it in the heart, but on occasion instead of feeling happy, we feel afraid, we feel embarrassed, as if love were a sign or symptom of weakness, when it is anything but. How difficult it is for us to express to a brother or sister how much we love them, saying it up front and looking them in the eye.

Manifesting it to our parents, children, husband or wife, or any of our loved ones, should be constant, because when we no longer have them, we would like to reverse time to tell them, and it is no longer possible. So we must not let another day go by without doing so, shouting it, hugging them like it's the last day of our lives. What are you waiting for? Do not stop, enjoy it, live it, discover the love born within that will make you feel that our only obligation as human beings is to be happy.

We must raise awareness of the future that awaits the generations to come. Make it very simple exercise that will give you amazing results.

For a moment imagine yourself as a fetus, pay attention to your surroundings and observe how every day, people are becoming less conscious.

The principles become excuses, the smiles are fading, and being cordial between people is a nuisance. We destroy our universe each second with new inventions, that although at the time we benefit from, we do not consider the side effects they can cause. It is logical that when taking a little time to imagine and seeing all these results, you would not like at all the idea of being born and living in a world with such problems.

I am sure that after this exercise you will be ready to take action on what for many years we have heard: Plant a tree, don't waste water, recycle, respect your neighbors and their spaces, give a helping hand to the youth so that their path is easier and safer, telling them your life experiences. They are the future of this beautiful universe, give a smile as it is a tool God has given you and is priceless, but with it you can brighten the lives of others opening different doors for yourself to achieve unexpected success.

Something very important: Practice the exercise of being honest with yourself.

I call it exercise because it takes time to achieve the practice of honesty and to make it part of our daily life, to achieve the result of being a better person, with a deep spiritual peace, and being away from depression and sadness.

Bad habits are easy to assimilate, but the good ones we find more difficult for several reasons.

God needs to hear that you are grateful for the gifts you receive. Thank the Universe for all the things that it gives you every minute, every second, including those that you consider to be negative. Leave them in the past as well as the people who have hurt you, because these are only experiences lived that need not hold space in your heart, occupying a place where you should keep only positive things.

It'll be on you if you do not learn from your experiences you will continue making the same mistakes! Although the future is uncertain, it should always be full of positive plans and successful projects, you just have to pay close attention to the present, as its name says it all, it is a gift, live it and enjoy it to the fullest, every moment.

I will tell you a story that is more than a simple motivational narration. It's a great reminder and a great lesson.

In a big city there was an ordinary man who always lived upset with life, continually complaining about the things that happened and never would thank the universe or the universal being for all he received.

One evening, while walking the universal being appeared before him, the creator of all things visible and invisible, and said; "My son, you spend your whole life complaining about what happens to you and never give thanks for the good things. Every day you ask for more believing it will make you happy. You ask for a bigger house, a new car and so on, the truth is I got tired of hearing this, therefore I have decided to grant you the last three wishes of your life and you must think clearly what you want, for I repeat, you will never have the opportunity to ask for anything else, for the rest of your life."

The man, without thinking for a second, made his first request. "The first I want is a new wife, young, beautiful and intelligent, for the one I have is tired and does not understand me."

The universal being asked; "Are you sure? Remember that you only have three wishes and nothing more, so you must be very sure of what you ask." The man replied that he was completely sure. Before this, the universal being declared: "Granted!"

The man continued on his way back home imagining what he would find when he arrived home. A large crowd surrounded his house, he walked to the door and realized that there was a coffin and that there his wife rested in peace, his heart began to beat heavily, he saw his daughter holding her newborn baby and her husband held her, comforting her for the pain that was happening. The young woman told her father, "Dad, my mother has left us. My son will not have a grandmother who will caress him and to tell him stories as my grandmother did with me."

The man began to feel bad, and later heard his own parents mourn the death of their daughter in law while saying; "Our poor son, how will he continue his life without the help of this great woman, who was an example of a person, always concerned about their children, home and her husband."

Then the man felt worse because he recognized that this was true. There were also coworkers of his wife, who also mourned her death and commented that she was a great woman. Her work was always on time, she was a very good friend and knew she was a great mother, always concerned about her children and working overtime to support her husband with college expenses.

In her free time she would look for new recipes to cook for her husband and surprise him with delicious dishes. The man began to feel like he was chocking, tears were streaming down his cheeks nonstop, knowing that all this was nothing more than the truth. With that, he ran out of the house seeking the Universal Being to beg him to return to him his wife and ask for forgiveness for his awful wish.

The Universal Being presented himself again before him and asked; "Are you sure of what you ask? Remember that after this wish is granted, you will only have one more wish." The man said; "I am aware of that, but certainly I want my wife back, because I realize that there will never be another woman like her." Having said all this, his wish was granted. At the same time the Universal Being asked if he was ready to ask for his last wish, to which he replied that not yet, because this time he would be more careful when making his wish. Ten years had passed and one evening, while walking again in the park, the Universal Being made himself present and after greeting the man asked; "What happened? You allowed a long time to pass and have not made your last wish." The man replied," You're absolutely right, but I actually thought of a thousand things to ask for, for example, I thought of asking for a lot of money, but if I had it, it would not ensure my health and if I were to become ill I would not be able to enjoy it."

"I also thought of asking for a lot of power, but it also does not assure my wellbeing or that of my family's, so I could not reach a decision.

Could I ask for your help to choose something that would really be good for me?"

The Universal Being smiled and said; "If I help you decide, remember that it would be as granting you another wish, therefore you could not ask for anything more." The man replied, "You're right", and inclined his head looking very thoughtful.

The Universal Being felt compassion for him and said: "I know that after asking for your previous wishes you learned a lesson, and thereafter you've been a great husband and a great father, but mostly an extraordinary human being."

"You have worked with your community, supporting your temple and more, and the best of all is that every day you're a better person. That's why I'll reward you by giving you the opportunity to ask for what every human being should ask for."

"First, every morning, you should give thanks for all that you receive daily, for opening your eyes to the universe, breathing and above all, to be alive to continue on your way. Only in exchange to tell you what you must ask for, you must promise to go through life preaching, so that way everyone learns what they really should ask for every day, having given thanks for what has already been received. What you should ask for is happiness, but not just for you, but for the world, because when you have happiness, you have everything.

"Friends, this story teaches us without a shadow of a doubt, that the only thing we should ask for each day is to be happy."

CHAPTER 27

Quotes, Thoughts and Phrases That Have Impacted My Life

"Even if I knew that my days would be over after my next birthday, I would still celebrate it in a big way."

- Mark Mounier's.

"Praying when I'm in trouble brings peace to my soul. But praying at all times, gives peace and joy to my life"

- Mark Mounier's

"I learned to love, accept, tolerate and respect others, when I realized I was imperfect myself"

- Mark Mounier's

"When I was a young boy I thought I knew what love was all about, but it was years after I married my wife, that I knew the great power of love"

- Mark Mounier's

"After many times of failing I learned that it wasn't the end, but it's the practice that makes me successful"

- Mark Mounier's

"Inspiration only exists if you dream, work and go for it"

- Mark Mounier's

"When you judge your partner, you will never get to truly love them"

- Mark Mounier's

"Being worried today makes me unhappy and look older than I would be in the future."

- Mark Mounier's

"All I want for this Christmas is to be with you, dad."

- Mark Angelo Moreno.

"You are number one on my list."

- Victoria Cecille Moreno.

I BEG YOU HEART

"Heart I beg you not to let me walk the uncertain path of this life without being sensitive to the pain and needs of those who pass my way. I pray that you do not deny me the force to always think positive, and even in the absence of that force, to never lose faith. Be true not only with myself but with the entire world and never lie to win the admiration of the people and get a false recognition. If life gives me wealth, never let me forget those who at the time of need have been with me and even more, never let me forget the needy. If during my history, life gives me triumphs never let me lose the simplicity without ever appearing weak. I ask the universe to gift me the sensitivity of common sense. Understanding that every human being is worthy of having their own opinions and thoughts without believing that if they think differently than me they're giving me their back. And to not despair over failure, to remember that failures are learning experiences to definitely achieve success. I beg you to help me always forgive because it is a sign of a happy and complete human being. And that pride is definitely a sign of an empty and unhappy being. If you give me success and one day in the same way on this path of life decide to take it away, give me the wisdom to understand that success is ephemeral but my faith and love for you are infinite! Do not let me forget to love my neighbor as I do myself and especially, Lord allow me to continue taking your hand for the rest of my life, as I have done so to this day!"

Mark Mounier's

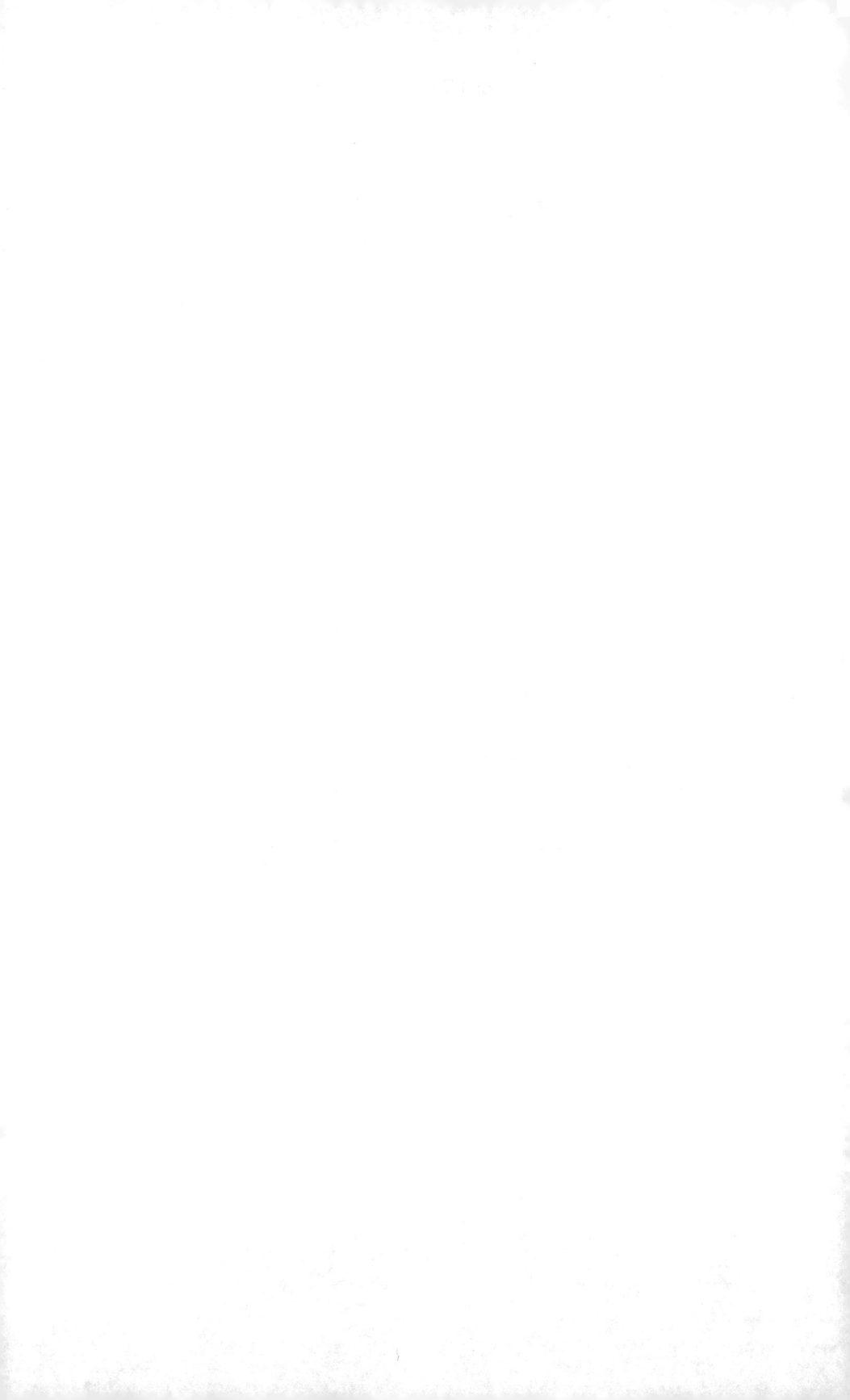

FAREWELL

"This has been a beautiful experience and I give thanks to the Universal Being for allowing me to fulfill it and to share it with all of you."

"In it I have poured not only my knowledge but also my heart, best wishes and love."

To all the people who in one way or another helped me with the realization of this book, I thank you infinitely: To my family for their unconditional support and for understanding my occasional absence in their lives, while doing this project.

Special thanks to two professionals and great human beings, for being accomplices in this project of mine, Attorney Cesar Cedillo; I love you friend, and Mr. Carlos Vargas, one of the best musicians I've heard in my life, for his collaboration in this project from 'A to Z', not only for supporting me with his music, his talent and his recording studio, but for sharing with me his knowledge to enrich this book.

I won't say goodbye, but until very soon, as we are already working on our future project, which I am sure will be of great interest to you.

Love you all, your friend,

Mark Mounier's.

DEAR BROTHER MARK

Only time and the years have given me the ability to understand, or rather, to comprehend how lucky I have been to have so many brothers as I have, with weaknesses and virtues, with different forms of thinking and feeling, but you know? I would not change anyone for any other, just the way you are I love you each and every one of you.

Today I refer to you especially, because the occasion calls for it.

I want you to know I'm proud of you. You grew up with me as the youngest of my brothers, and like no one else I've seen how much you've succeeded. How step by step you forged goals and succeeded in each of them.

I once commented that no money or gold is enough to buy a brother. You can have friends, good friends, but it so happens that life teaches you that suddenly they may cease to be, but instead, a brother will forever be…Always brothers.

I wish you the greatest success in this book that you've done with so much vision and I dedicate the poem MY GREAT GIFTS, born from my heart, my soul and inspiration that God gifted me.

God bless you!

Your brother,

Gustavo

MY GREATEST GIFTS

When I opened my eyes to life
And gave my first steps
I saw myself surrounded by so many gifts.
They were only mine:
They were my siblings.
And I asked heaven,
what did I do to deserve so much?
Because life would give me
Handfuls of… smiles,
laughter and occasional sorrow.
They were my siblings,
playing on the patio,
climbing the tree,
eating a mango
in that house we inhabited
in that house
were we loved each other.
And as time passes
how I remember you:
You, the youngest
taking my hand
feeling my support
feeling me as a brother.
Today I can tell you
looking into your eyes
how much I admire you
and even more.
How much I love you.

Gustavo Moreno

www.ingramcontent.com/pod-product-compliance
Lightning Source LLC
Chambersburg PA
CBHW061305280526
45784CB00002B/907